The role of hospital consultants in clinical directorates

The Synchromesh Report

Edited by
Anthony Hopkins
Director, Research Unit,
Royal College of Physicians

1993

ROYAL COLLEGE OF PHYSICIANS OF LONDON
in association with
THE KING'S FUND

Acknowledgements

The chapters in this book and the discussion which follow are based upon a workshop organised by the Research Unit of the Royal College of Physicians and the King's Fund, London. The papers on which the chapters are based were revised and edited in the light of the discussion, which was tape-recorded and edited. Roger Williams and Peter Mumford helped organise the programme.

The Research Unit of the Royal College of Physicians is supported by generous grants from the Wolfson Foundation, the Welton Foundation, the King's Fund, other donations to the College's Appeal Fund, and by the Department of Health.

The editor is grateful to Janice Bowman for her help in organising the workshop, and to Fiona Shipley for secretarial services.

Royal College of Physicians of London
11 St Andrews Place, London NW1 4LE

Registered Charity No. 210508

Typeset by Dan-Set Graphics, Telford, Shropshire
Printed in Great Britain by Cathedral Print Services Ltd, Salisbury

Participants

*Indicates authors of papers

Helen Bowers *Elderly Services Manager, Queen Alexandra Hospital, Cosham, Portsmouth, Hants PO6 3LY*

Christopher Burns-Cox *Consultant Physician, Frenchay Healthcare Trust, Directorate of Medicine, Frenchay Hospital, Frenchay Park Road, Bristol BS16 1LE*

*__Cyril Chantler__ *Professor of Paediatric Nephrology, Department of Paediatric Nephrology, Evelina Childrens Hospital, Guy's Hospital, Guy's Tower, 9th Floor, St Thomas Street, London SE1 9RT*

Derek R Cullen *Consultant Physician and RCP Regional Adviser, Royal Hallamshire Hospital, Glossop Road, Sheffield S10 2JF*

*__Wendy Darby__ *Business Manager, Department of Geriatrics, The Ipswich Hospital, Heath Road Wing, Ipswich IP4 5PD*

Sir Terence English *Consultant Cardiothoracic Surgeon, Papworth Hospital, Papworth Everard, Cambridge CM3 8RE*

Andrew Frank *Clinical Director, Orthopaedics, Rheumatology and Rehabilitation, Northwick Park Hospital, Watford Road, Harrow, Middlesex HA1 3UJ*

Stephen Griffin *Director of Personnel, St James's University Hospital, Becket Street, Leeds LS9 7TF*

Colin A Hardisty *Consultant Physician, Northern General Hospital, Herries Road, Sheffield S5 7AU*

*__Anthony Hopkins__ *Director, Research Unit, Royal College of Physicians, 11 St Andrews Place, London NW1 4LE*

John R Horsley *Consultant Physician, Ormskirk and District General Hospital, Wigan Road, Ormskirk L39 2AZ*

Adrian Jennings *Senior Registrar, Northern General Hospital, Sheffield S17 4LY*

Roland T Jung *Clinical Director of General Medicine, Ninewells Hospital and Medical School, Dundee, Scotland*

*__Robert J Maxwell__ *Chief Executive and Secretary, King Edward's Hospital Fund for London, 14 Palace Court, London W2 4HT*

__David Mitchell__ *Clinical Director for Medicine, St Mary's Unit, Praed Street, London W2 1NY*

*__Bryan Moore-Smith__ *Consultant in Geriatric Medicine, Department of Geriatrics, The Ipswich Hospital, Heath Road Wing, Ipswich IP4 5PD*

*__Judith Riley__ *Fellow in Management Education, King's Fund College, 2 Palace Court, London W2 4HS*

__Martin N Rossor__ *Clinical Director for Medical Specialties, St Mary's Hospital, Praed Street, London W2 1NY*

__Michael Rudolf__ *Consultant Physician, Ealing Hospital, Uxbridge Road, Southall, Middlesex UB1 3HW*

*__David Scott__ *Consultant in Rheumatology, St Bartholomew's Hospital, West Smithfield, London EC1A 7BE. Present address: Reader in Rheumatology, King's College School of Medicine and Dentistry, Bessemer Road, London SE5 9PJ*

*__Martin P Severs__ *Consultant Geriatrician (formerly General Manager), Elderly Services (Acute), Queen Alexandra Hospital, Cosham, Portsmouth, Hants PO6 3LY*

*__Jenny Stephany__ *Senior Business Manager, Directorate of Medicine, Medical Specialty Services, St Mary's Unit, Praed Street, London W2 1NY*

__Robert B Tattersall__ *Professor of Clinical Diabetes, University Hospital, Queen's Medical Centre, Nottingham NG7 2UH*

*__David A Walker__ *Consultant Physician, Department of Medicine for the Elderly, St Luke's Hospital, Crosland Moor, Huddersfield HD4 4RQ*

__Tony White__ *Orchard Farm, Jarmany Hill, Barton St David, Somerton, Somerset TA11 6DA*

__Ian R Williams__ *The Walton Centre for Neurology and Neurosurgery, Walton Hospital, Rice Lane, Liverpool L9 1AE*

*__Roger Williams CBE__ *Second Vice-President, Royal College of Physicians and Director, Institute of Liver Studies, King's College School of Medicine and Dentistry, Bessemer Road, London SE5 9PJ*

__Eve Wiltshaw__ *Director of Clinical Services, The Royal Marsden Hospital, Fulham Road, London SE3 6JJ*

Foreword

by **Sir Duncan Nichol** CBE
Chief Executive, National Health Service
and
Professor Leslie Turnberg
President, Royal College of Physicians

The sub-title of this report—The Synchromesh Report—is a reference to the Cogwheel Report of 1967 which introduced the concept of management by consensus with health professionals. It is generally agreed that the resulting diffusion of responsibility and accountability was not a tremendous success, and the institution of general management following the Griffiths Enquiry in 1983 has led to more focused management and a clearer sense of direction for those who provide health care. Hospital consultants and hospital managers must work together in order to provide the best quality clinical care within the available resources. There are obvious potential tensions in the relationship. For example, managers may feel that individual consultants, in their wish to provide the best possible care for the patients in their specialty, are distorting the overall provision of services to the local community. On the other hand, some consultants may feel that their managers do not fully understand the clinical imperative of their work with patients. None the less, the work of doctors and managers must always be in gear—hence The Synchromesh Report.

We welcome this book which explores one relatively popular method of involving doctors in management—the clinical directorate. The concept that a clinical team which provides one particular aspect of service or services within a hospital, should be responsible for managing its own resources and for developing plans within the overall institutional strategy is an attractive one. Nonetheless, there are difficulties which are not clearly resolved. Examples include the conflict that a clinical director has in continuing his or her own clinical work and research and yet sparing adequate time to manage the directorate, and the potential tensions between the aspiration of individual directorates and the strategy of the institution as a whole. We welcome the initiative of the Research Unit of the Royal College of Physicians and the King's Fund in sponsoring the workshop on which this book is based, and we are confident that all who read it will draw from it ideas on how they can best develop their own work within NHS hospitals.

Editor's note

For non-UK readers, a 'session' of a consultant's contract with a trust or health authority is half a day.

The subtitle of this report—the Synchromesh Report—is a reference to an earlier governmental report on the organisation of medical work in hospitals, commonly referred to as the Cogwheel Report, on account of its cover design of gears.[1] It was a standing joke at the time (1967) that the gears, as drawn, could not turn.

Contents

1 | Historical background: where have clinical directorates come from and what is their purpose?

Cyril Chantler

Professor of Paediatric Nephrology, Guy's and St Thomas's Medical and Dental School, London

As a result of an earlier reorganisation of the National Health Service in 1974, the Board of Governors of Guy's Hospital in London was abolished. A *district* management team accountable to an *area* health authority was established with a requirement to operate within the confines of consensus management, as outlined in the Cogwheel Report.[1]

In 1976 the then Labour government introduced the concept of cash limits to public expenditure. These were tightened within the discipline of cash planning by the Conservative government that came to office in 1978. These changes were combined with the application of the recommendations of the Resource Allocation Working Party (RAWP),[2] which resulted in a progressive transfer of resources from the overprovided health regions in the southern part of England to the underprovided north, mediated by an allocation formula based on the numbers of population adjusted in various ways according to standardised mortality, social deprivation and so on. The further application of RAWP subregionally resulted in a transfer of resources from inner London to elsewhere in the Thames regions.

The *area* health authorities were themselves abolished in 1982. Guy's health district and the Lewisham health district formed a new authority. The responsibility for operational management of services was divided into three units: Guy's Hospital, Lewisham Hospital and Priority/Community Care Services. The management teams involved in each were accountable to the new *district* health authority. The new authority conducted a strategic review following which it determined on a transfer of resources from acute hospital care to the community services, thereby foreshadowing the wider changes introduced in the NHS and Community Care Act 1990.[3] General management was introduced following the NHS management inquiry conducted by Sir Roy Griffiths in 1983.[4,5] The cumulative effects of these policies involved a radical reduction in the funding available for Guy's Hospital.

Demand and resources

The demand for resources according to the needs for clinical care was until 1978 expressed by the professionals working in the service, particularly the doctors. These demands had been met by allocation by the Department of Health of new resources on a year by year basis. The unwritten philosophy was that the health professionals would determine the allocation of resources, accepting the need for careful husbandry, whilst the government would endeavour to meet all reasonable demands. The application of cash planning led to a widening gap between what was available and what was thought to be needed. Health professionals argued that the government was not keeping its side of the agreement by providing more resources as demand rose; conversely, the government felt that the health professionals, by continually seeking more resources and enlisting the help of the media to emphasise their demands, were not acting responsibly. The conflict spread to individual hospitals, with doctors and administrators constantly criticising one another. The problems at Guy's were particularly acute because of the reduction in available finance described above. By 1983 it had become clear that the infrastructure of the hospital was being neglected because the administrators did not feel able to maintain the fabric of the institution at the expense of a reduction in clinical activity. Whether all activity was efficient was never asked.

The lack of cohesion in management was well demonstrated in 1984 when the district management team decided to close more than 100 beds in order to save money. During the two months following closure, throughput in the hospital increased to a level higher than in the same two months of the previous year. Guy's Hospital thus had the dubious distinction of being the first London hospital to spend more money by closing beds.

Clinicians in management

Some clinicians at Guy's had been watching with interest the experiment of involving clinicians in a decentralised operational management structure at the Johns Hopkins Hospital in Baltimore from 1972. They persuaded the district management team to visit the Johns Hopkins, and they too were impressed with what they saw. It was therefore agreed that a similar management structure would be started at Guy's in April 1985 on an experimental basis. The essential nature of the contract was that clinicians would take a dominant responsibility for the operational management of Guy's; in return for the authority to influence the allocation of resources, they would accept responsibility and accountability. This accountability included acceptance of financial accountability.

Guy's Hospital 1985–1988 and thereafter

The task confronting the new management team should not be underestimated. There was a considerable backlog of necessary capital expenditure, amounting to many millions of pounds, which had to be met immediately. Examples included repairs to the cooling system in the tower block, a new air-conditioning system for the operating theatres, new lifts, a new telephone exchange and much necessary refurbishment. The new management team was also required to accept a reduction of £8 million per annum in revenue over three years, about 15% of total available revenue each year. This formidable task was more or less achieved, the hospital balancing its budget, and meeting its savings target. In spite of this reduction in revenue, throughput of patients improved. Perhaps what was most impressive was the changing and improved relationship between different health professionals and between health professionals and administrators.

Principles of the involvement of clinicians in management

Philosophy

There has to be an acceptance by clinicians of the reality of cash limits; within them, all have the ethical responsibility to ensure that resources are spent wisely to ensure effectiveness and efficiency. Where money is limited, profligacy in the care of one patient may lead to the denial of care for another. There must be constant attention to improving efficiency in economic terms and ensuring the effectiveness of treatment to produce the best outcome. These considerations link into the national initiatives in resource management and clinical audit.

Professional and management accountability

It is important to distinguish between professional and management accountability. Clinicians are *professionally* accountable to their patients and to their professional colleagues. Although the remuneration of the clinician in the National Health Service comes from central government, it can be legitimately represented as coming from the patient, from whom it is raised by taxation. It is therefore right that all staff should be accountable *managerially* for their use of resources within the institution for which they work. Thus, in the Guy's system, all staff are managerially accountable, often to individuals who come from a different professional background. However, the bounds of professional accountability have not been changed; nurses, for example, are still professionally accountable to nurses. In essence, the chief nursing officer of Guy's is responsible for managing nursing rather than nurses.

Responsibility, authority and decentralisation

The essence of decentralisation is to improve the involvement of all staff in the operational management of their service. Responsibility and authority must be coterminous and commensurate. There is a tendency for central administration to decentralise responsibility, but not financial authority or operational authority. Conversely, clinicians in a decentralised management structure wish to acquire authority, but without responsibility and accountability. These issues need to be discussed and worked through if the system is to be effective.

Management can be broadly divided into two parts: guidance (strategy) and delivery (operational management). The task of a clinical directorate is mainly operational management, but the clinical director leading and representing the clinical group should have a voice in strategy. The hospital management board at Guy's is chaired by a medical director who is a clinician; it is made up of all the clinical directors and functional managers.

Part-time clinical commitment

If clinicians are to be involved in management, they must be allowed to fulfil this responsibility on a part-time basis. If they are required to devote a great deal of time to their management function they will cease to be clinicians, their unique perspective as clinicians will no longer be contributing to the management task, and their capability to lead will be inhibited. However, if they are to fulfil the responsibilities of a clinical director on a part-time basis, they must be prepared to share this responsibility with other members of the management team, recognising that their role is management, not administration. They need to be supported by able business managers. The emphasis is on a team approach. The basic team comprises a doctor, a business manager and a nurse manager, working together. The profession of the leader of the group does not need to be specified, though the tendency has been, at least initially, for this role to be filled by the doctor.

There is a difference between management and administration. Doctors may have difficulty in getting involved in management because they take on tasks of administration; these are themselves professional tasks and designated members of the team should be responsible for them. Management has been said to be about doing the right things, whereas administration is about doing things right. However, everybody, especially the professionals in hospitals, should be involved in the management process.

Information systems

It is often argued that one cannot manage without sophisticated information systems. This is not true, although it is the case that the better the information the better the management function will be. Staff costs account for about 72% of expenditure in most hospitals, so control of staff costs is a basic discipline required for financial stability. Likewise, it is most important in improving efficiency to ensure that each member of staff is as productive as possible. Information systems should be designed to improve first the running of the clinical directorate and the provision of clinical services. The necessary management information should be derived from these functions.

The most important lesson that has been learnt from the introduction of clinical management at Guy's is the importance of getting the structure right and the need to change attitudes of all those concerned. If these aspects are not properly discussed and debated, no information system is likely to benefit the hospital.

Clinical directorates are based on the concept of team work between all staff; to be successful they depend on the breaking down of professional barriers. Our experience suggests there are four points that are important in the introduction of this concept.

- Professional and management accountability are discrete and should not be confused.
- Decentralisation should be encouraged, producing a broad, flat management structure for operational purposes, with clear definition of responsibilities and authority (which must be commensurate) and accountability.

- The commitment of professionals involved in general management at clinical directorate level should be part-time so that they can continue to fulfil their professional responsibilities. Team work must be encouraged; the leadership of the team does not need to be defined in advance but does need to be determined.
- Adequate information systems should be introduced. They should be determined primarily by the clinical needs of the directorate; the data should, however, be structured to fulfil management requirements.

Conclusion

The main task now is to allow the changes in the National Health Service to bed in and to allow sufficient time to develop the initiatives that have been started. Although we have to operate within cash limits, balancing the budget is simply a prerequisite for the management of the National Health Service, not the reason for creating it which is still to improve the health of the nation and the quality of the clinical care given to patients.

DISCUSSION

Roger Williams: Can you describe how the present pattern of management is different from that at the start? Has the system developed in response to problems? Or have there been no problems?

Cyril Chantler: There certainly have been problems. There were internal and external concerns over the application for trust status. The central management team, instead of concentrating on the task of delivering the service, became very involved in strategy and guidance, because we did not have a district health authority or board of governors at that time to develop a strategy. The team may have taken their eye off the ball a little in regard to operational management.

One problem has centred around the number of clinical directorates or, putting it another way, the size of the team that provides the operational focus. We had 14 or 15 directorates, which seemed to me to be a number with which I could cope, but we are now experimenting with a rather larger group of about 24. We developed a coherent team from that number. Other hospitals have decided on smaller groups of four to six.

John Horsley: It may be important to get the numbers right early on, and it is probably better to start with a small rather than a large number of directorates. If you do it the other way round, you end up having to deprive people of some responsibilities to which they have grown accustomed after a few years.

Have you found ways of avoiding the need for consultants to devote too much time to management? Doctors really only retain their credibility in management by retaining clinical credibility.

Cyril Chantler: Doctors must understand what their role is in a management team. As the clinical director within a clinical directorate, or as the medical director of the whole team, if you do only the things you are truly there to do, they should not, I think, put an unworkable burden on either your clinical practice or your research. If you become involved in the details of administration, certainly your practice and research will suffer. You need good administrative support, and you have to trust it. But once you have built up a team relationship, being a clinical or overall medical director should not really require the sort of time that people fear. I hear of people spending three or four sessions a week on being a clinical director; that seems unreasonable. When I was chairman of our management board, which was a bigger job than being a clinical director, I genuinely did not spend more than that time on the task. I think two half days, split at different times during the week, should be enough time to perform well as a clinical director.

One must be beware of management consultants who come in with no experience of hospital or medical practice. There is no received wisdom that they can use to advise you. You have to look internally rather than externally for your solutions. The size and number of directorates will depend very much on local circumstances. I do not think there is any magic figure or number that you can determine. The solution also depends on the people you have and who is prepared and interested in clinical management.

Terence English: What led you to expand the number from about 14 to 24 directorates? How is this experiment working?

Cyril Chantler: Some directorates at Guy's found it easier to work in this way. Paediatricians have tended to operate over the years as a group within Guy's, sorting out their differences behind closed doors and then having a coherent voice in the hospital as a whole. So having five subgroups in paediatrics, each with its own budget, and managing its own part of the clinical service based on a ward and outpatients service, has not proved to be a problem.

With other directorates, that concept proved to be less easily applied, and having one director representing the whole of a specialty caused considerable unhappiness amongst other consultant members of the team. They felt that they were not able to manage their own service in the way they wished. They wanted to organise their service and to have a voice at the top table of the strategic group for the hospital. So now a number of what had previously been subdirectorates have become directorates in their own right. However, they share the same business manager with other directorates within the broad area of practice in which they operate.

This is why we have the present number of directorates. It is too soon to say whether we have the right number. Twenty-four is a huge span to control, and there is a real risk that in such circumstances the whole structure can begin to break apart, rather like Italy before Garibaldi. There has to be a central cohesion to hospital policy. You cannot have everybody doing their own thing. We shall just have to wait and see how our present system works.

An alternative approach is to have, say, about six directorates as at St Thomas's Hospital. This seems to be working quite well. Six group directors spend a fair amount of time on their management activities but relate to subdirectorates, each with its own budget; the group directors represent the subdirectorates in the hospital policy group.

The fundamental task of the Guy's management board is to make the *operational* management of the hospital as good as it can be; because that is decentralised, each of the clinical directors is responsible for the operational day by day management of his or her particular service. They come together on the hospital management board to make sure that their policies are not in conflict, and to contribute, where appropriate, to advice concerning the strategy of the institution as a whole.

The *strategic* responsibility rests with the board of governors or the directors on the trust board. Their basic task is the development of strategy. They should get involved in operational issues only where necessary. Operational management and strategy must be clearly seen to be the major tasks of two separate parts of the organisation.

I am critical of the way the financial function in the NHS has developed over the past five years. Our own finance department finds it difficult to provide clinical directorates with accurate, concise budget statements month by month, linked to proper analysis of clinical activity and so on. I believe the reason for this is not that it is impossible but that central finance practices in the NHS are not accustomed to such a necessary function, have no experience of doing it, fear what would happen if they introduced it, and have simply not put the necessary enthusiasm into it. I now know that such budgeting is possible because the medical school, of which I am now dean, has introduced such a system over the past year.

If you are clinical director of paediatrics, it should be possible to calculate the amount of your contract income. Deducted from it first should be your directorate's share of the overhead costs of the hospital, which are easily analysed. Then should be debited agreed top slicing, which reflects the hospital's business plan on a year by year basis. Everybody has contributed to the discussion to develop the business plan, but finally central management has determined the items for the common good for future development that will be provided from common income. The remainder of the contract income then devolves to the directorates. They buy back, from other parts of the hospital or from outside, the services they require to fulfil their responsibilities.

This seems to me a straightforward system. The computer systems and software are, of course, already available. As long as you work on a year by year business planning process, there should be no problem about making sure that hospital policy is followed through. The trust board is responsible for ensuring a coherent management policy and function for the hospital.

Eve Wiltshaw: Suppose you want to change the emphasis of your hospital from, say, medicine to surgery; you want to change the numbers of surgeons in relation to the numbers of physicians. How does a trust board or central management do that when its directorates are wanting to 'do their own thing'? Who has the resources for medical and nursing manpower? Do you lose the flexibility to change your hospital radically if you give budgets to the directorates in the way you have described?

Cyril Chantler: We tackle this by reviewing each year the expenditure of different directorates and pulling money out of their budgets for the next financial year to return to the centre. This is then reallocated to the same or other directorates according to need as determined after full discussion by the hospital management board. This is a year by year business planning process, which is how other organisations operate.

Purchasing and contracting are the new influences now. Budgets will be determined more and more by the demands of customers, so there really has to be a system for reallocating money. We have done it in the medical school—since we also have purchasers, the research councils, the university funding council, students' fees and so forth—by giving out each year two budget figures. One is the actual budget the department will get. The other is an indicative budget which reflects the business strategy of the hospital as a whole. The departmental task is to produce a business plan to bring them into line. This will mean savings for those whose indicative budget is less than their actual budget. As that money returns to the centre, so it will be redistributed to those whose indicative budget is greater than their actual budget. I cannot see any reason why a similar system could not apply within a hospital.

I know there are problems over flexibility in redeploying staff, but that is not true of all groups of staff and, managed with some sensibility and over a period of time, change is certainly possible.

Colin Hardisty: Clinical directorates have now been in place for about seven and a half years at Guy's. How successful do you feel this system of management has been?

Cyril Chantler: I have no doubt that the experiment has been successful. It brought us through an extremely difficult period. We were able to save large sums of money and to begin to push money into some essential expenditure that had been neglected. Our new systems of management also improved enormously the relationships between different professional staff. You do not hear people at Guy's now referring to 'management' as if its members were some separate species, because now everybody is involved. You do hear people referring to the centre of the hospital, but that is not in terms of any professional function; there are doctors at the centre as well as accountants and administrators, resulting in a much more healthy and enjoyable working atmosphere.

There are several reasons why our changes have not been totally successful, some of which I have already noted. The controversy over trust status knocked us off line; there have been staff changes in the administrative and finance organisation, so new groups of people had to learn and strengthen the organisation. We could have moved faster if we had had better and more enthusiastic management for accounting, and there is no reason, in my view, why we should not have. It seems to be in the nature of public sector accountants to distrust these ways of working.

The finance officer of the medical school, who has now been with us for about 24 months, came from the private sector; he could not understand why we had not been doing many of the things that for the previous decade I had been told were difficult if not impossible to do. For example, I had been told that a management information system would take years to develop. He asked why we did not buy one. He said it would cost £40,000 and he knew one that would 'do the trick'. He had a different perception of what was required. I am not trying to disparage public accountancy, but it seems to have a different agenda.

We have not been as successful as we could have been but we are all learning as we go along, and it is important that we share our new knowledge.

2 | Diary of a clinical director

David Scott
Consultant in Rheumatology, St Bartholomew's Hospital, London

I was clinical director of a combined medical and surgical directorate of linked specialties (rheumatology and orthopaedics) for two years until October 1992. The surgical component was predominant, although I am a physician. The setting is a major London teaching hospital group with both clinical and academic involvement. The clinical directorate structure was established in 1990 and I was appointed in August of that year, but for my first 12 months virtually nothing happened. The substructure of the directorate was incomplete, financial information was limited, and there was relatively little pressure involved.

Structure of the directorate

There were initially six consultant surgeons with varying sessional commitments, and three physicians. The physicians also took part in acute general medicine; two of them were partly or entirely funded by the medical college. The directorate included: eight intermediate grade junior surgical staff, six house surgeons, two intermediate grade junior medical staff and three house physicians, also involved in acute general medical admissions; eight medical secretaries, two senior clerical/administrative staff, a senior nurse and a service manager; nursing staff for three wards and two outpatient clinics. Our annual budget was £2 million. There was also support from a financial adviser and an assistant general manager who worked in association with a number of other directorates. Service provision is based on two units, each with a different atmosphere and environment, separated by three miles of busy city traffic.

Setting the scene

In 1991 the directorate was asked to make a 5% saving on its budget. It became obvious that the only way to achieve a reduction in costs was to reduce staff. It also became evident that one of the issues was the contribution of some staff to the workload. After discussions, two surgeons reduced their sessions though continuing within the unit in highly individualised arrangements, one through the NHS and the other through the medical college. This left a hole in the cover for emergency admissions.

The diary

The diary begins on 1 May 1992. The teaching group had just become a shadow trust with the introduction of a trust board and an external chairman. One surgeon had just withdrawn from the duty rota for acute admissions and a second was on the point of doing so. A new service manager also started at the beginning of May. The diary covers the next ten weeks. Rather than give a day by day account, I record a week by week summary of the main events.

Some events are fixed each month; for example, the clinical policy group responsible for all directorates in both units met for a whole morning on the third Wednesday of each month. I was also a member of the human resources committee (a subgroup of the clinical policy group dealing with staff matters). However, most meetings were *ad hoc* arrangements.

First two weeks of May

I start the month quietly with Bank Holiday Monday. New arrangements have been made for the acute surgical cover, each of the two hospitals covering acute admissions on alternate days. This is necessary because of changes in the working arrangements of two consultant surgeons.

I have numerous telephone calls from the accident and emergency unit about the changes in the acute surgical cover.

I have a telephone conversation with the dean about academic development of the surgical specialty in the light of the change in consultant staff. I recommend the appointment of a new senior lecturer.

I am summoned one lunchtime to an urgent meeting with the deputy head of all clinical services about the acute surgical cover.

I hold a meeting of some members of the directorate, attended by some of my consultant colleagues and the senior managers. There are discussions about surgical cover, the proposed new consultant appointment and the academic development of the surgical specialty.

I am summoned from my clinic to another urgent meeting about acute surgical cover.

At the end of the second week I am in Maastricht in Holland for a scientific meeting of my specialty, considering measures of disease severity in joint disorders.

Third week of May

I start the week by seeing the professor of surgery about academic developments in the surgical specialty. He recommends an immediate NHS consultant surgical appointment, a transfer of other consultant sessions to the medical college, and an external application for support for a new academic non-clinical senior lecturer with additional support staff.

I see the college secretary to get further advice on academic surgical developments.

I brief our new service manager on the directorate.

There is an urgent meeting of the human resources committee about junior doctors' hours; the Department of Health requires that their hours be reduced to 72 per week, which creates problems over out of hours cover.

Last week of May

There is a change of surgeon to whom I principally relate on surgical matters within the directorate.

The clinical policy group meets to discuss junior doctors' hours and the poor contracting position. A special group is set up to discuss arrangements for surgical cover within the directorate.

At a further meeting of the human resources committee we discuss the unresolved problem of junior doctors' hours.

First week of June

There is an emergency meeting about junior doctors' hours after the institution has taken external advice on its position. A potential solution is explored with the junior representative.

I see the dean with an academic plan for the surgical component of the directorate which will have links with the medical component. Help is promised. I attend the board of studies in surgery for the same purpose.

Second week of June

There is an emergency meeting to try and resolve the continuing problem of acute surgical cover.

Third week of June

I see the chief executive of the shadow trust about the appointment of a new NHS consultant surgeon and the academic development of the surgical specialty.

The clinical policy group meeting concentrates on the poor financial position of the shadow trust. We are told that block contracts are reduced by 10%; for surgical specialties this means a 20% reduction for non-acute work owing to virement (replacing non-acute work by emergency admissions within a contract). There is a need to maximise work on long waiting cases funded by the waiting list initiative, and on extracontractual referrals.

We try to resolve the continuing problem of acute surgical cover at another emergency meeting.

I see a senior academic physician about problems in developing the academic links with the surgical specialty.

Fourth week of June

The deputy senior nurse of the institution sees me to discuss interactions with the directorate's senior nurse, which are not ideal.

End of June and beginning of July

I see one of the surgeons who reduced his sessions in order to rationalise his work schedule, and explain to him the need to focus on extracontractual referrals.

I speak again to the senior academic physician about problems in the academic arrangements for the directorate.

There is a meeting with the new director of general surgery to resolve problems about the job description for the proposed new NHS surgeon.

I see the other surgeon who has reorganised his sessions through the medical college for a specialist service, and explain to him about the need to fund this through extracontractual referrals.

I have a planning dinner with the senior nurse and service manager.

The Kings' Fund Commission report for London becomes available. I read it and reflect on the development of services in the next few years in our institution.

I arrange for all the medical specialist cases to be admitted to the cheaper of the two hospitals, a plan that has not yet been fulfilled.

Second week of July

I see the senior surgeon in the directorate to explain the planning needed to meet the new contracting arrangements. This is followed by a more detailed discussion with all the surgeons. There are some difficulties in explaining about the reduction in block contracts and the need to focus on long wait cases.

Secretarial chaos develops when temporary secretaries are disallowed by central management owing to the financial position.

I visit another institution outside the NHS to try and obtain extracontractual referrals.

I see one of the surgeons who has reduced his sessions, to resolve issues relating to his contract with the college and to reinforce the advice about extracontractual referrals.

Third week of July

I see the college secretary to try and resolve issues of contracts with a consultant surgeon.

I have another meeting with the college secretary to try and resolve the academic development of the surgical unit and its interaction with the medical unit.

I attend a meeting of the human resources committee which considers the problem of reducing junior doctors' hours to 72 per week by the beginning of August. This is largely resolved. The financial status of the shadow trust remains a cause for concern.

A successful meeting with the director of general surgery leads to the completion of a job description for a new consultant post and its advertisement.

A member of the administrative staff tells me that a member of the NHS executive seconded to our institution has suggested that the Tomlinson report will make bleak reading for us.

My problems as a clinical director

If I had realised the problems and difficulties in being a clinical director at present, I would have had serious reservations about taking the post. It was extremely hard work, the problems were difficult and partially insoluble, there was little advice or guidance on what to do, and there were tensions with colleagues.

The implication that money would follow the patients after the NHS reforms proved to be totally incorrect. There is no shortage of patients, merely a shortage of contracts. The main problems have been an unknown base for block contracts, continual changes with rules for waiting list initiative work, lack of funds for outpatient work, difficulty in defining an extracontractual referral, and a constant stream of reports and recommendations about London teaching hospitals. There was also a local problem of attempting to run a service across two sites, with decreasing staff and reductions in junior doctors' hours.

I had no training at all for being a clinical director. No one ever told me what to do, how to arrange the directorate, what the institution was trying to achieve, or what would constitute good plans for the future. Central management proved to be unstructured. Important decisions were made at the last minute and often by default.

What happened later

Several things took place in September and October, many of them surprising. The main events were: a new consultant surgeon was appointed and took up his post at an early date; the delivery of surgical care improved and problems about emergency cover were resolved; activity on the medical side of the directorate declined; I was invited to move to another teaching hospital and accepted this invitation. An accident and emergency consultant also moved to another institution. If the opportunity ever arose again to be a clinical director, I should decline. I do not regret the experience, but do not wish to repeat it.

DISCUSSION

Roger Williams: How much time would you assess you spent per week on directorate matters, taking you away from rheumatology?
David Scott: In an average week it was about a session at the most. I did not have an enormous amount to do for much of the time that I was clinical director. In May, June and July last year, the period covered by my diary, events took a somewhat different turn, and I think about half of my time in May was involved in meetings. There are times when things get difficult, and then the pressure eases. The difficulty is to predict when those times are going to arise. I had no reason to suspect that May would be a particularly awkward month, but several problems arrived together.
Michael Rudolf: From your diary and hearing you talk about what happened, I am sure there is not a person here who does not sympathise with you. One is aware of an incessant demand to have

meetings, and more urgent meetings. I feel strongly that when agreeing to become a clinical director you should lay down ground rules about your availability to come to urgent meetings at short notice. One's full-time managerial colleagues, who do nothing but have ad hoc meetings, may find it difficult to accept that busy clinicians might not be quite so free to do so. When I took up my clinical directorate I insisted that only at set times during the week would I be available for ad hoc meetings. Many problems that appear to be urgent can often be dealt with later at a more convenient time.

David Scott: It is difficult when colleagues in the accident and emergency department are insisting that a particular matter must be discussed at length. Central management often seemed to want 'endless' discussions about the topics I have mentioned. It is difficult to limit discussion and yet maintain close working relationships with one's clinical and managerial colleagues.

Cyril Chantler: There are occasions when one just has to leave outpatients, but many matters are not so urgent that they cannot be dealt with outside normal clinical times. You can say 'I'm sorry, I can't come at three o'clock, I'm in outpatients. What about eight o'clock tomorrow morning?' That usually has the effect of determining whether a meeting really is urgent. However, as unit general manager, I was in a more powerful position than a clinical director. I am aware of clinical needs and I did not lightly ask people to break into their clinical practice; for example, many problems can be solved over the telephone without meetings. If there is some consensus about the areas for discussion before a meeting, the business will be speedy. Good papers written and circulated before a meeting are much better than having a non-structured discussion. We need to pay attention to our management of time.

Colin Hardisty: It seems that you lacked support from senior colleagues. Surely, when you run into difficulties of the type you describe, central management should take over; either the director of all clinical services or the chief executive should be sorting out such problems after a reasonable period of time. Do you feel that there was a lack of support, that problems were just handed down to you as clinical director and everybody washed their hands of them, and you were rushing around trying to sort them out?

David Scott: Everyone from the dean to the chief executive of the shadow trust was extremely supportive and very helpful whenever I saw them. I think they had the same difficulty. None of us really knows the rules about how best to manage change. I do not think they knew any better than I did how we should change the

structure, and perhaps the passage of time is sometimes what is
needed. Within the NHS we may not yet have the correct organisational philosophy to deal with change. So I do not think it was lack
of support; it was just that none of us quite realised the right way to
go. The original problems have largely settled. Now my colleagues
have to cope with a separate set of difficulties. The constant
change of the past two years has caught most of us out.

Eve Wiltshaw: David Scott's problems may have in part arisen
because he started without a proper job description, and did not
know to whom and for what he was accountable.

Roger Williams: The definition in your contract of your exact role
and responsibilities must be important, because in that way you
can ensure that the time you spend working as a clinical director is
appropriate for your continuing clinical work. At my hospital we
have one doctor termed 'clinical director', who is on the executive
board. At other hospitals this doctor may be called 'director of
clinical services'. How do the clinicians in charge of individual
directorates relate to this other doctor, who perhaps may be more
involved in central management and may be more powerful or
influential?

David Scott: Shall I answer for Bart's first of all? Nineteen directorates met together as a clinical policy group once a month,
which was attended by the dean, the chief executive and the director of clinical services, who also had a deputy. One could telephone the director of clinical services and discuss issues at any
time, but of course he had a lot of different pressures coming his
way. His job is to make strategic decisions within a small working
executive. We never really sorted out together who should make a
decision about what.

Cyril Chantler: It is important to understand the organisation of
management that you are putting into place, and that everybody
else involved understands it as well as possible before you start. If
you do not understand the organisation, when faced with the need
to change, a need which will continue, you will not understand the
structure you have in place to cope with the difficulties. This is certainly a lesson that I have learned.

The role of the clinical directors, and therefore directors of all
clinical services, should be understood by everybody, both above
and below them, when the organisation is set up. In my role as
chairman of the hospital management board and unit manager, I
was accountable to the district general manager of the district
health authority for the operational function of Guy's Hospital. It
is important that the doctors, ie the clinical directors, know who

has the authority either to help reach a decision or to go to the health authority with strategic plans. Let us take as an example the issue of junior hospital doctors' hours. This is such a complicated issue and involves so much radical change throughout the hospital, both between different professions and between different clinical directorates, that I do not see how you can approach such a problem piecemeal from the bottom. Such a problem really has to be dealt with at the centre, linking into the decentralised structure. It cannot be initiated by the decentralised structure. The solution to a problem may be difficult to achieve, but the means of approaching that solution ought to be clear.

Andrew Frank: Cyril Chantler divides up strategy and operational management and gives the impression that strategy is somebody else's affair. In reality you have to operate in line with your strategy.

Cyril Chantler: You cannot separate operational management and strategy; they impinge one on the other. I have always felt it to be important to have a clear strategy in any organisation; otherwise how do you make decisions on a day to day basis? I put more emphasis on a partial division of responsibility. The particular task for the clinical directorates is operational management, though they contribute to the strategy. The task for the trust board is more strategic, but obviously there are certain operational issues that concern them as well.

Roland Jung: I have been clinical director for general medicine for about two years. What surprised me when I started was how little knowledge our business manager had of personnel matters as they affect the medical profession—extra duty hours and so on. Dr Scott, did you have any help from your business manager in sorting out these matters?

David Scott: Yes, but there are complications because of the rotational nature of many posts. For example, the orthopaedic senior registrar rotation is so complicated that anyone has difficulty in understanding it. But people have been as helpful as they can. We have had tremendous changes in the staff of the human resources department in our institution over the past three or four years. It has lost many of the people who had been there for many years, and that has resulted in ignorance of the history of the organisation. The general strategy in regard to junior doctors' hours was fine: the limit was to be 72 hours per week from 1 August 1992 but problems in implementing it have been the difficulty.

Cyril Chantler: The whole process of management is new to many. We have a view that, because colleagues are called managers, they must have experience of management. Many of them do not; their experience is no greater than yours. Many also come from a culture of administration rather than management.

Robert Tattersall: I was clinical director of medicine until I resigned about six months ago. I sympathise with Dr Scott. I had two principal problems, especially the calls to urgent meetings, for example about quality standards in outpatients, which meant I had to leave my patients waiting in outpatients. But I also had moral problems. For example, I had data showing that the nursing levels on the general medical wards had been inadequate over the preceding five years. I was then told that I had to cut 2% off the nursing budget. I simply refused and, pointing to these figures, said that we needed more nurses, not fewer. This really comes back to what Cyril Chantler said. I believe that the quality of the service is all-important. I was stuck between trying to maintain the quality of the service and reporting upwards in the organisation to people who clearly did not share this belief. I found it an intolerable position.

Cyril Chantler: I was told by senior nurse management at Guy's on more than one occasion, quoting nurse dependency figures, that more nurses were required for a service. I accepted this and argued much as you did. I cannot talk about the particular circumstances on the wards about which you spoke. What I do know is that I was misled on that. There is an Audit Commission report on the value of nursing which makes interesting reading.[6] It shows a wide variation around the country in the nurse staffing levels for similar functions with similar outcomes. Changes that are now being made in nursing skills provide at least as good a service as before and are much less expensive. It has to do with how you organise the whole ward. At what time are the clinical activities taking place? How long is the overlap between shifts? What is the level of night staffing? How many state registered general nurses are there as opposed to nursing assistants? We introduced at Guy's a group of night practitioner nurses who respond first to certain calls from the wards, rather than the junior doctors. This is one of a number of examples of changes in practice.

We have to consider also the cost effectiveness of the service and constantly to search for better and cheaper ways of doing things. There is plenty of scope for experimentation in the role of the casualty department, accident and emergency department—drop-in clinic, if you like—in the provision of emergency care in inner cities. So I think we should encourage experimentation, but at the top of the agenda should be the quality of the care that is provided, and that needs to be audited at all stages.

We need to concentrate on doing simple things well. It is easy, when one is involved in clinical management or the management of any organisation, to be attracted by the broad strategy and by radical and exciting change, but we should be concerned about how long people wait, about operations being cancelled at the last minute, and about how we can facilitate the transfer of patients from the hospital into a caring environment when hospital care is no longer required. These sorts of operational issues can only be addressed in a decentralised fashion, because it is the people providing the care who have to come up with designing and managing solutions.

3 | Benefits of clinical directorates

David Walker
*Consultant Physician, Department of Medicine for the Elderly,
St Luke's Hospital, Huddersfield*

The objectives for the clinical directorate in general medicine at the Huddersfield Royal Infirmary, which includes geriatrics, dermatology, rheumatology, haematology and genito-urinary medicine, were largely based on the White Paper of 1989: 'to ensure that hospital consultants—whose decisions effectively commit substantial sums of money—are involved in the management of hospitals; are given responsibility for the use of resources; and are encouraged to use those resources more effectively'.[7]

It was and is argued that, if consultants assume some or all of these extra responsibilities, certain benefits will follow. For example, decentralised decision making by those closest to patients should be faster and more responsive to the ever changing needs of users of health services. Health professionals, who know a lot about the health care business, should be the ideal people to plan the delivery of high quality services. More effective budgetary control should in theory follow. Health services, managed more effectively, will be determined by contracts agreed with purchasers (health authorities and general practitioner fundholders) according to population and individual health needs.

Consultants are a loose-knit peer group. They are highly individual and independent. They work hard and take pride in their excellence. They are champions of the doctor-patient relationship. Their energy contributes to continuous improvements in the delivery of health services. But there is also a darker side. Their hard work can lead to overcommitment, with little spare time to learn new skills. In a situation of scarce resources, an energetic, powerful consultant may 'win' resources at the expense of some other service. The sanctity of the doctor–patient relationship may undermine other loyalties to their organisation (specialty, hospital, district or the NHS).

If change is to occur, these strengths and weaknesses must be recognised. A number of paradoxes need thorough discussion, for example:

- Working very hard and yet finding time to devote to new activities
- Continuing to do what doctors do best and yet developing new skills
- Safeguarding the doctor–patient relationship and yet caring for the organisation
- Searching for excellence and yet being prudent with resources
- Potential conflicts between independence, isolation, and feeling trapped by work
- Winning and losing local battles for resources and yet cooperating with other professionals.

Many of these paradoxes have yet to be fully resolved but the fact that they have been recognised means we are no longer at the beginning of the process of change. This cultural shift has been supported by management through clinical directorates at Huddersfield since April 1990. There are at present four directorates: medicine, surgery, children/women, and the providers of services to the main clinical services (anaesthetics, radiology, pathology, pharmacy, physiotherapy, occupational therapy, ECG, domestics, catering, laundry, CSSD, works, porters). Each clinical directorate contains doctors, nurses, medical secretaries, ward clerks and medical records clerks. Each directorate has a board made up of three consultants, a business manager and a nurse manager. One of the consultants is chairman of the directorate and reports to the hospital general manager. The range of service activity of clinical directorates is determined by contracts with purchasers. In theory the delivery of service is determined by internal agreements.

A number of tasks facilitated this process of change. In the implementation of a 72-hour junior doctor working week a great deal of time was required before agreement was reached amongst general physicians and geriatricians. Full junior cross-cover and registrar rotations followed. The business planning cycle, developing and implementing the objectives of the directorate within the framework of the overall hospital strategy, has been a powerful vehicle in which consultants have examined their current position and evaluated their future. The Patient's Charter has been another important stimulus to change.[8]

Resource management has not been taken up as rapidly as it should have been. Clinicians must recognise the need to control cost and realign or develop services according to contracts. Central resource management has resulted in some changes. Spare capacity generated by one directorate was taken up by another and an extra geriatric ward was opened.

Another factor which has assisted change is a regular monthly meeting of all consultants in medical subspecialties. This has been supplemented by three meetings per year covering topics such as team building, business planning, working toward trust status, management skills, audit, information management, computing and other topics. Consultants come together to talk about what they do, to share facilities, and so on. The problem of junior doctors' hours has been a plague on our houses, but it has led general internal medicine and geriatrics to cross-cover for the first time in Huddersfield and talk together about how they might share services. The eleven consultants have also considered their capital priorities, and how best to use their beds in response to the report of the Audit Commission.[9] The major gain has been the move from an isolationist type of culture within the hospital to a cooperative venture in which we all win or lose together rather than separately. Clinical directorates must avoid being isolationist and merely perpetuating what has happened in the past but in a new form. They must relate to other directorates, to providers and to senior managers, and contribute to the overall framework.

There remains the relationship with central management. When clinical directors are ready, will there be devolvement of budgets and decision making? Senior management has found it difficult to let go, especially financially. If we are to be involved in management, be given responsibility for the use of resources and make more effective use of those resources, we should have access to them in the first instance; but that has not happened yet.

We must consider our relationships with provider departments. By this, I mean the services we buy from our colleagues in X-ray, pathology, and so on. The notion of them surviving on their contracts is still new. It is difficult to progress without a lot of discussion and reassurance, much as we have done in relationship with our external purchasers. Management tends to get in our way when we have direct conversations with those who purchase our services, and those from whom we purchase internal services.

My last point is about training. The clinical director is an agent of and for change; he or she needs support to bring about these changes, and is likely to need training in the necessary skills. Part of the learning process has been to stop assuming that what we do now is good or adequate. During my first 18 months as clinical director I was less than happy. I felt somewhat isolated. I felt 'got at' to a certain extent. But I have had some help and some training. I have also had to improve some of my interpersonal skills.

DISCUSSION

Roger Williams: One matter that has been raised is the internal contracting system. Various clinical directorates in my hospital are sending bills, or statements as to what they are expecting from other clinical directorates in this coming year. The liver unit has been leading the way in sending out bills, and I have had a series of letters back from my colleagues asking why they are being charged and whether there is not a simpler way. It involves much more administrative work, of course, and in that the clinical director clearly has a role.

David Walker: This is an explicit way of trying to achieve quality financial accountability and interdisciplinary teamwork. I accept that there will be more paperwork. We are, however, helped by an internal contracts manager, who relates closely to the managers of the individual directorates.

Ian Williams: At my hospital, we have internal contracts only for services for which we think contracts are important in managing the quality or extent of the service. For example, the chemical pathology laboratories and the X-ray department would be expected to write a contract with each clinical service but we would not expect one clinical service to write a contract with another clinical service: their interaction would be based on a 'gentleman's agreement'. We did not feel that it would improve patient care if bits of paper were passing round the hospital as bills for clinical interactions.

Derek Cullen: I should like to explore the interface between geriatric medicine and general medicine in which David Walker is obviously involved. In my region, one often finds the two disciplines in different directorates and they do not seem to want to get together, yet the fusion of the two would have obvious advantages for both. One fundholder in Leicester will not purchase either general medicine or geriatric medicine unless they fuse. Are there other ways if the fundholders do not address the issue?

David Walker: We have maintained the old Cogwheel set of committees[1] alongside the directorate structure: the 11 medical consultants meet once a month round a table, whereas the directorate structure involves just three consultants who work as an executive for the medical division. The necessity for people to do business has been important, and this did not happen before the creation

of medical directorates. The medical division previously was con-
vened about once every six months if there was something to talk
about. But as clinical director I have encouraged people to meet
on a regular basis. They are committed to one hour a month.
Three times a year we have speakers from outside to discuss matters of common interest.

The outside pressures that have made us build our relationships
were the problem of junior doctors' hours, and the need for cus-
tomer service, providing for their needs and preferences. This
notion is still in its infancy. No doubt, as the purchasers and the
patients and their relatives become more powerful, patients will
want to see the doctor who will service their needs best—whether
that is a respiratory physician, a cardiologist or a diabetologist.

Christopher Burns-Cox: I think that to some extent the happiness
of an institution depends on preempting anxieties; keeping the
Cogwheel divisions[1] until they die naturally, if that is what is to happen, is a good tactic. We still have a division of medicine. It does
very little, but it is there to give professional advice to the people
who run the directorates. It is a happy relationship. It is atrophy-
ing, but at least people feel the clinical director is not the only
physician who can express views. This is one way of achieving a
balance.

Another way is to have regular meetings of physicians. In our
hospital, senior registrars and consultants meet twice a week for an
hour at half-past eight in the morning. That is a business meeting
which I run, with a lot of business items, and it works well.

Cyril Chantler: For the Cogwheel divisions[1] to continue absolutely
unaltered while a clinical directorate is introduced alongside is
potentially dangerous. A Cogwheel division of medicine could
become like a 'government in exile'. Since the division does not
actually carry authority, their advice could be disruptive. What
gives you authority when you give advice, it seems to me, is if you
carry responsibility and you are accountable for it. Having said
that, there is an absolute requirement for all staff in the institution
to have easy procedures for their views to be made known to the
management of the hospital, and those views should be taken into
account. To advise and consult is absolutely imperative in all management. So there has to be a medical committee where the views
of the doctors can be presented, both to the directorate system
and to the board of governors of the trust or to the health authority. Within each specialty there also has to be a forum where the
doctors, both junior and senior, can meet and ensure that the clinical directors can receive their advice, and also discuss ways of

implementing directorate discussions relevant to their speciality. How you do it—whether you call it a Cogwheel division or something else—is an individual matter, but such systems must exist.

John Horsley: Does the clinical directorate system require a medical director or director of clinical services over it, or is that an unnecessary duplication, particularly in smaller hospitals? I can see that in a large hospital like Guy's there is a need for someone senior to coordinate the individual directorates, but in the smaller hospitals the interpersonal workings are obviously very important and it may not be appropriate to have one clinician in charge.

Christopher Burns-Cox: When we set up the directorates 18 months ago, we were all concerned that managers might want to 'divide and rule'. We were aware that, if we did not have a medical director or a director of clinical services whom we knew we could totally trust, there would be another potential source of paranoia in the system. We therefore insisted that the medical director be chosen from amongst the clinical directors. So she is one of us, as well as being the medical director on the trust board.

Roger Williams: How often does the medical committee, including all the consultants, meet at Guy's Hospital?

Cyril Chantler: The medical and dental committee meets four times a year. The agenda always includes a report from the medical director (the director of clinical services), who then answers questions. When we first set it up I was rather hoping I could get all the clinical directors along as well, so that the whole medical and dental committee could raise points with them. It mostly turned out that I was there on my own, answering questions. The medical committee also set up a standing committee during the difficult time when trust status was under discussion. This met monthly to inquire into any aspect of the activities of the trust, and people took that seriously. Within the directorates, of course, members meet. Most specialties meet regularly with the director of clinical services.

Andrew Frank: I am not certain to what extent it is unusual, but at Northwick Park we will shortly have consultants in two different trusts working on the same site. The acute services unit will be one trust, while the other is the pre-existing community services trust. The physicians in geriatric medicine and the psychiatrists are part of the community services unit. Clinicians from both trusts need to meet together on the same campus, so we have retained the medical committee on which every consultant sits by right. That has been a useful talking shop and an alternative meeting of clinical directors, other non-clinical management colleagues and the consultant body as a whole. I agree that one has to have an alternative meeting to the directorate structure, even if it is only every one to two months.

4 | Models of organisational support for clinical directors

Bryan Moore-Smith *Consultant in Geriatric Medicine*
Wendy Darby *Business Manager*
Department of Geriatrics, The Ipswich Hospital

In 1990 the Institute of Health Services Management stated that 'any hospital doctor needs to have an understanding of and basic competence in management. Even if a consultant takes on no special role in management, the normal clinical role increasingly demands some sophistication in managing people, using financial and clinical information, managing time and communicating well.'[10]

These attributes are essential in those playing an active role in clinical management. If they are to maintain an effective clinical role as well they require assistance in their management capacity. They also require training.

The Institute of Health Services Management document describes three organisational models for clinical management:

1. The consultant coordinator
In this model (Fig. 1) the unit general manager retains managerial control and accountability for professional and managerial hierarchies, and is in contract with the consultant coordinator to monitor and coordinate consultant colleagues and staff in a clinical unit/team. The consultant coordinator does not hold the budget for the total clinical service and is not responsible for the management or performance of other team members. Teams are not corporate bodies and cannot be held accountable for budgets or performance as a group.

2. The clinical general manager
In this model (Fig. 2) the operational management of clinical services is delegated to clinical general managers who may be of any professional background. Medical/management relationships are conducted through medical representatives but there are no explicit contracts between consultants and general managers.

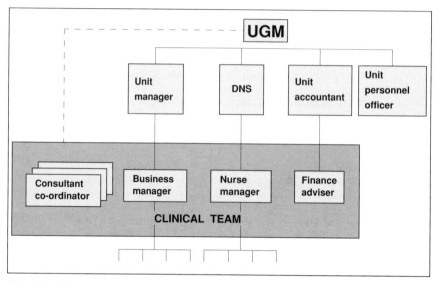

Fig. 1 The consultant coordinator organisational model (DNS, director of nursing services; UGM, unit general manager). Reproduced with permission from reference 10.

3. *The consultant manager (the clinical director)*
In this model (Fig. 3) the operational management of the clinical service team is highly decentralised. The unit general manager is in contract with consultant managers who coordinate consultant colleagues and manage clinical staff.

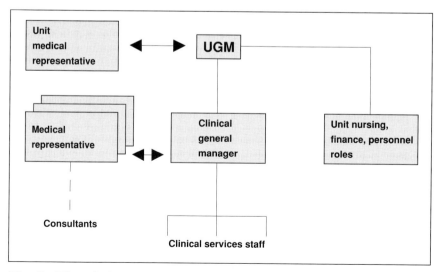

Fig. 2 The clinical general manager organisational model. Reproduced with permission from reference 10.

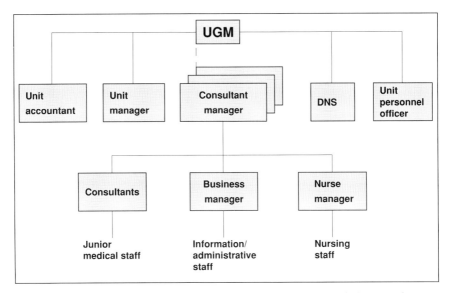

Fig. 3 The consultant manager organisational model. Based on a Figure from reference 10.

They hold the total budget for staff and services within their clinical unit. They are also responsible for all aspects of day to day management, recruitment and selection, staff appraisal and staff development. Here the unit general manager's role changes from manager of all operational services to negotiator and coordinator of clinical contracts.

Management and specialist roles at unit level need redefining to support clinical units rather than manage professional hierarchies; they cannot be held accountable for the work of their professional equivalents in the clinical unit.

We believe that each of these models represents a stage in the development of the role of clinicians in management. The first option, the consultant coordinator, appears to stand by the old style of hospital management and does not follow the principle of devolved ownership and responsibility, whereas the clinical general manager model could be seen to be representing an 'idealist' solution, and presumes that there has been a massive shift in cultural attitudes both within the hospital and within the individual professions. Our experience is of the third option, the consultant manager (more commonly called clinical director). We describe more fully our experiences with this model.

The usual structure of this model is the formation of several directorates responsible for their own specialty, eg elderly medicine, general surgery. The directorate is managed by the clinical service team which consists of a clinical director (consultant), a nurse manager and a business manager. Each has specific areas of responsibility and expertise, and acts as adviser and support for the others.

In order to function at all, a clinical director must receive support in the form of accurate and timely information, assistance in the day to day management of the staff of the directorate, and advice in unfamiliar areas of expertise, not infrequently personnel matters. The main forms of support are provided by three specific categories of people:

• Managerial: provided by the business manager and the nurse manager
• Information: provided by the business manager and the nurse manager
• Advisory: in the form of external support from personnel, and finance departments, for example.

Managerial support

It is impossible for the clinical director to retain a continuing clinical workload without being able to delegate managerial responsibilities for nursing and clinical staff, and in some directorates for other professionals such as laboratory technicians and radiographers. Other health professionals, such as physiotherapists, occupational therapists and speech therapists, have for the most part their own management structure, a point of potential difficulty in itself with respect to the needs of a directorate. The clinical director must be able to delegate the solutions of day to day management issues of non-medical staff while retaining final control when necessary.

The nurse manager has the largest day to day management role, with a wide span of managerial responsibilities for establishment, the consideration of skill mix, acting as professional head and adviser, dealing with disciplinary matters, setting standards and counselling staff. For the most part, the nurse manager's professional advice on nursing matters to the clinical director is likely to be accepted, within the overall resource constraints of the nursing budget (but see page 22).

The business manager is generally managerially responsible for the administrative and clerical staff.

The clinical director has the responsibility of managing his consultant colleagues and the junior medical staff. Much can be achieved by the mutual sharing of budgetary and performance information and peer review, without the need for 'confrontational intervention'. In more difficult circumstances, the clinical director may prove to lack managerial training and experience. Issues such as performance related pay might in the future prove contentious if implementation were devolved to directorate level.

All these managerial roles are crucial to the smooth and efficient running of a directorate. Any managerial problem that arises in any area can be discussed at meetings of the directorate team, which may prove an invaluable support and give the opportunity for innovative suggestions and solutions.

Information support

Without good, reliable and timely information, sensible decisions are difficult to reach. The computer revolution has made possible the production and manipulation of vast quantities of data which by their very abundance may only serve to heap obscurity on confusion.

The business manager's role is crucial here, first as a collecting and sifting point for centrally and locally produced figures and statistics and, more important, to condense and simplify the information into a clear, accurate and timely user friendly form. Local information produced to central dictates may be almost useless for day to day management purposes. If no action results from information provided, it may be assumed that its value is low.

Second, he or she has to be responsible for obtaining the correct information. In an era of rapid cultural change, factual information is an essential aid to assist that change to take place; without information, arguments are conducted in a welter of supposition and personal opinion.

Information support will be needed in the following principal areas:

Budgets

It is important to devolve the budgets to as low a management level as possible; this means down to ward level and individual consultant level, monitored by the business manager. If you do this, people start to realise that they are actually committing financial resources. Everyone has the same information and shares it. They can see what their colleagues are doing and then they start to ask questions as to why certain colleagues do certain things and incur certain costs. The answers to these can sometimes be comfortable, sometimes uncomfortable, but they are often illuminating.

The key to budgetary control is the monthly review of budget performance by the clinical service team. The business manager must be capable of and responsible for analysing the budget statements, identifying areas of under- and over-spending, and recommending any necessary action to the directorate team. In addition to this, monthly budget and activity data packs are distributed by the business manager to members of the clinical service team, senior medical staff and ward managers.

These packs include analysis and comparison of trends as well as breakdowns and comparisons of drugs expenditure, X-ray usage etc. This can often be a powerful tool in expenditure and activity control, and has so far been met with interest, helping to develop an understanding of different methods of working between individuals.

The drug budget in many directorates is the most intractable to change. Apart from price inflation, prescribing habits may be hard to alter, and the pressure from pharmaceutical firms hard for some to resist. Support may be obtained from hospital or departmental formularies, as well as from appropriate guidelines for the treatment of common conditions.

Contract monitoring

Management is aware that successful contract performance is now its primary aim for the hospital, but this is much less apparent to clinical staff and not infrequently leads to mutual incomprehension.

There is a worry in my hospital that the management—and here again one is falling into the trap of talking about 'the management' as opposed to the clinicians, which perhaps says something about the state of development of clinical directorates in our particular hospital—tends to be driven by the need to fulfil contracts. The clinicians tend to take the view that their purpose is to treat patients. There is obviously a dichotomy there which is difficult to bridge.

Monthly contract statements and their variance from expected outcomes are an important support tool for clinical directors. It may be difficult to discuss with clinical colleagues the reasons for variance in activity or outcome, and troublesome decisions may need to be made.

Activity analysis

Departmental activity figures, including numbers of patients treated (both inpatients and outpatients), inpatient lengths of stay, procedures carried out and prescribing costs, all require thorough analysis and can provide useful managerial information on emerging trends.

Coding and diagnosis related groups

No directorate can work effectively unless the case mix is known. Accuracy of clinical coding is most important and should be seen as a major responsibility of the directorate. The hospital central information department should offer a vital support role.

Manpower

The establishment is usually historical, but changes can be effected by variations in skill mix. This is perhaps easier in the nursing field because of the larger budget. Change within the medical manpower budget is more difficult, but central initiatives such as the recent requirement for shorter working hours for junior doctors should be seen as an opportunity to enhance the quality of service and provide better training.

Business planning

The support of all disciplines is required in the preparation of a business plan. Their different requirements need to be evaluated in terms of the opportunities they present and the problems they expose for the directorate as a whole. A business plan written without multidisciplinary involvement is likely to founder. Consideration must also be given to the shape of the overall strategy for the hospital within which a directorate's plan must be contained.

In a staff intensive organisation, the business plan offers the appropriate means of identifying future staffing requirements as well as the buildings and facilities that may be needed. All these factors will call for evidence from the relevant disciplines and agencies.

Service data

Most directorates need the help of the service departments such as pathology, diagnostic imaging, operating theatres and remedial professions. Many hospitals are moving towards devolving the budgets for such services to directorates. The pattern of service provided and the cost implications will need to be agreed. The monitoring of such contracts then falls to the business manager as part of the information support to the clinical director.

Advisory support

Personnel department

Although the nurse manager is primarily responsible for the nursing staff and the nursing budget, in this particular model he or she is accountable to and subject to individual performance review by the clinical director, as indeed is the business manager. In the final analysis, serious disciplinary matters within the directorate fall to the clinical director for resolution. This is not a field in which many doctors have expertise.

There are potential difficulties of individual performance review,[11] already part of the contract of the nurse manager and business manager. This is not yet part of the consultant contract, although one can see that things might go that way. What would happen to distinction awards, for instance, if the distinction award system persists in some guise?

When disciplinary procedures are invoked the clinical director may have to chair any necessary hearings. In such circumstances the advice of the personnel department is essential. Provided the disciplinary procedures have been properly established and the course of action is fully understood, the hearings have a logic of their own, but appropriate personnel support is imperative.

Finance department

Few doctors have financial training, and budget statements initially lack clarity to the uninitiated. While the method of providing information can be learnt fairly easily, problems arise if it becomes apparent that the budget, for whatever reason, is not going to balance. In some circumstances advice from the finance department on how to address the situation can provide vital support, especially if working relationships can be built up. Presentation of a draft budget proposal is usually part of the clinical director's job description. The assistance in this of the business manager, nurse manager and finance department is most important, although in current financial circumstances it is more likely that a directorate will be presented with a budget rather than be involved in its preparation together with central management. If a directorate's budget seems to be in balance it may be left to manage alone without support that could further benefit service to patients.

Clinical audit

The influence of clinical audit on contracting is potentially considerable. Audit informs the clinical director about opportunities for quality improvement of both process and outcome. As a management tool, audit may be valuable in ensuring that alterations, for instance, in treatment guidelines are properly costed, and that full cost/benefit calculations are carried out on new approaches rather than introduced on a tide of enthusiasm, simply because they appear to be a good idea. If the cost of change appears to be greater than a constrained budget will allow, audit may lead to other options being examined which may be more beneficial to patients and to costs than the original suggestion. Equally, if it can be shown that a higher quality outcome is obtained at greater cost, virement between budgets may be arranged to allow for this better opportunity, and to make a case for an enhanced budget in the next business plan.

The clinical service team within a directorate

One of the most useful sources of immediate advice and mutual support is the clinical service team—the clinical director, the business manager and the nurse manager—a small group all in direct contact with the everyday realities of running a complex organisation. Some teams meet fortnightly or monthly. Some involve all senior medical staff in team meetings, but other clinical directors meet with senior medical staff separately. There are points for or against either model but we have found that discussion in a small multidisciplinary group can be informal and unthreatening, and confidential issues can be discussed freely. Other staff can be coopted as required.

The clinical service team has regular weekly meetings involving the clinical director, the business manager and the nurse manager. The agendas are formulated by the business manager and cover a variety of subjects from pure information exchange on daily activity to strategic plans for future developments. Supporting this forum there are several other groups which meet separately. The ward sisters meet with the nurse manager, the business manager being in attendance. Consultants meet weekly with the clinical director and the business manager. One of these is attended on a quarterly basis by the business manager. Monthly meetings are held at ward level between the ward sister and the relevant consultants in order to discuss matters of mutual interest and concern. They are timed to occur immediately after the issue of the monthly budget statements by the business manager.

A multidisciplinary team advisory to the clinical service team of 7 to 9 people has been established. This meets in alternate months, depending on the business to be discussed; it proved extremely useful during the business planning process. Clinical service team members attend its meetings.

Conclusion

Adequate, appropriate organisational support is essential for efficient management. Authority and responsibility need to be devolved to clinical directorates if they are to work well.

Each member of staff has an essential role to play in the support of an organisation, and each person must accept responsibility for his or her actions. As they rise up the career ladder, the responsibility and authority and the need for the ability to make difficult decisions become greater. There needs to be a high degree of trust in working relationships.

Support for a clinical director, without which his or her tasks would be impossible, must be widely based. Individual directorates need to evolve a model that suits their particular requirements which themselves are likely to change and evolve.

5 | Role of the business manager in clinical directorates

Jenny Stephany
Senior Business Manager, Directorate of Medicine,
St Mary's Unit, London

The tasks of a business manager can be separated into the two broad categories 'care and maintenance' and 'change and development'.

'Care and maintenance' includes staff management, operational management and financial management, and the management of information and communication within and outside the directorate. It is mainly to do with routine matters and is rooted either in the past or in current 'fire fighting'. 'Change and development' includes information analysis to assist strategic and business planning, maintenance of relationships with the purchasers of care, clinical audit, and bringing forward new developments. These elements require planning and a longer time frame for achievement. In an average week in our large clinical directorate, approximately 60% of time is spent on care and maintenance and 40% on change and development.

In my experience there has been a mismatch between the theory that decision making is decentralised and the continuing reality that key decisions continue to be taken either by professional groups or by central management. There has also been a lack of shared priorities agreed between central management and the directorate, giving rise to unrealistic expectations and failure to deliver results. Work is often duplicated, or left undone, as responsibility for moving tasks forward is left unclear. There has also been a gap between the needs of the directorate for information and the ability of the organisation to provide it. Examples include the failure to ensure that the information is reliable and to provide information that can be used for management purposes within the directorate.

There has also been confusion about the nature of the directorate support team and their roles and responsibilities, and about

the balance of centre/directorate loyalties. Examples include with-
holding information and outbreaks of 'professional tribalism'.

We have also experienced organisational pressures which
encourage 'fire fighting/reactive' responses rather than the development of new initiatives or different ways of delivering service.
An example is related to outpatients, where solving problems
piecemeal has been encouraged, rather than a radical consideration of the changing external demands and the impact on the service now required. All this is taking place against a backcloth of
continuing tension between pressures to reduce costs and improve
services.

The market in health care

The managed market encourages more explicit consideration of
alternative options for meeting health needs. Providers need to
respond faster to changes in demand for services and to become
more flexible and able to adjust capacity in line with changes in
demand, for example by managing elective work in different ways.
The business manager needs to help the clinical director to make
choices about the use of scarce resources. Both need to develop
analytic skills and to consider cheaper alternatives for fulfilling
their contracts. For example, a purchaser may develop a greater
range of residential and day patient care, reflecting different
patient dependencies.

The current emphasis on the views of users of health services is
likely to encourage providers to develop more 'patient friendly'
services than hitherto. It is probable that this will encourage all
staff to make suggestions for improvements in service delivery
throughout the organisation. In short, clinical directorates must
ensure that the organisation of service delivery is driven by the
users of health care, and the market. This is a shift in focus from a
service that the institution wishes to provide to one that the market
wants.

Central management and clinical directorates

The relationship between central management and the clinical
directorate needs to be designed to ensure that central management and central support departments have an enabling rather
than a constraining role. However, central management must
retain an arbitration function, necessary for strategic purposes.
Clinical directorates should be encouraged to be entrepreneurial,

imaginative, responsive to change in need, and flexible in patterns of service delivery. They should operate as autonomous business units with decisions made as close to the patient level as practicable. They should manage their resources either directly or via explicit internal and external contracts. They should focus effort on development and change, while continuing to ensure that quality and other standards are met. They should receive timely and reliable information to permit effective analysis for future planning and for monitoring the services they provide. They should ensure that the roles, responsibilities and accountabilities of all members of the directorate are clearly defined.

Roles and skills of the business manager

A number of roles can be identified, including:

- General manager of the directorate's business: the pivot who makes things happen, who ensures effective management of the directorate, who manages projects, who is in charge of day to day monitoring of the service provided, and who liaises with support departments.
- Marketing coordinator: the person who identifies opportunities, harnesses the 'sales force', and involves other staff in discussions on improvements to the services provided.
- Business analyst: the person who, in the context of resource constraint and external and internal opportunities, develops business plans and improvements in the use of resources.
- Change agent: the person who creates the climate to encourage appropriate change, and ensures effective management of the change process.
- Teacher: a person who helps explain the directorate's function and plans to other staff members, and who provides support, reassurance and encouragement to respond to the challenges presented.

In order to undertake these roles a range of skills is required:

- Basic management competence: including management of people, resources and information
- Personal effectiveness: ability to manage time, order priorities, analyse, delegate, organise and facilitate
- Interpersonal skills: including management of teams and professionals with credibility
- Skills in communication, negotiation, and management of change.

Conclusion

The business manager can add value to the directorate's clinical function by developing the role in ways that ensure a more effective linkage between the needs of purchasers and patients and the service delivered. The nature of management now is to support the clinical unit rather than to manage professional hierarchies. Providers who wish to survive in the turbulent environment of the 1990s will need to adapt to uncertainty and change.

The new post of business manager fulfils a number of roles. The first is to champion the directorate, to help its at present rather fragile structure to survive. There is an element of being a teacher, as we all learn about the new environment. There is also a general management function and a marketing function, but I think that the two key elements of the role relate to the analysis of problems and information and helping in change.

We learned from earlier discussion how it is possible to become submerged in detail and spend time rushing from one meeting to another. One contribution of the business manager is to help the directorate to focus more on proactive than on reactive management.

What does the business manager need to do well to succeed? There are some critical factors for success, and I cite first openness and trust, but credibility is important also. You need to be credible within the directorate. The consultants and other members of the directorate need to know that they can come and discuss problems in a constructive way.

It is also necessary for there to be a clarity of roles, particularly between the clinical director and the business manager, so that each is clear about who can add value in a particular situation, and duplication of effort can be avoided. Good communication is critical to success.

DISCUSSION (Chapters 4 and 5)

Roger Williams: The two preceding chapters have raised important matters concerning the relationship between the business manager and the clinical director. Does central management normally turn to the directorate's business manager for advice, since they are used to dealing with other managers and administrators, rather than to consultants who usually head the clinical directorate?

David Mitchell: You are right to raise the question of the relationship of the directorate's manager with central management. It relates to the incommensurate distribution between responsibility and authority, not only of the clinical directors but also of the business manager, particularly in a time of greatly constrained resources. Our trust board, and I expect all other trust boards, will be determined to work within their budgets. This raises tensions between the centre and the business manager. For instance, the business manager may wish to employ some agency staff just to keep the show on the road, but the centre may refuse on the basis that expenditure must be cut or jobs will have to be lost. That is just one example of the kind of tension that occurs.

There is often much discussion and duplication in the decision-making process. It is easy for a large amount of time to be wasted and for the roles of the business manager, the clinical director and central management to become blurred and confused.

When the centre want something done, in my experience they are equally likely to call me or my business manager; it depends on the issue.

Stephen Griffin: I agree with the point made about bringing clarity to management arrangements. Perhaps the second and more important issue which is starting to come out is that of accountability. Many of the problems between the trust board or senior management and clinical directors concern financial accountability. The issue about 'letting go' or devolvement is all very well if you let go of accountability as well, but in many cases you do not; the financial accountability remains firmly with the trust board and the chief executive.

Cyril Chantler: Budgets must be devolved to the level at which the costs are incurred. At Guy's Hospital we did not do that at first; we left it at clinical director level. But that might involve a number of different clinical teams—hopefully not single consultant teams—and you really have to devolve budgets to where the service is actually being provided, and where the contracts are to be negotiated. It does not seem to me possible to negotiate contracts on behalf of a clinical team without involving it, although I am sorry to say that that is happening and is causing chaos where I work.

Responsibility and authority need to be coterminous. The institution requires proper accountancy systems so that the centre can monitor what is going on. The centre's fear is that, by devolving responsibility and accountability, it will lose control and central management will pick up the bill at the end. But that is really a question first of confidence in colleagues, and second, of having in place accountancy and auditing systems to make sure that a problem is tackled before it begins to throw the whole institution off course.

Jenny Stephany: I think the challenge is to focus on the key role of the business manager. There is a real danger that the business manager becomes the dumping ground for whatever the organisation does not think needs to be dealt with at the centre. That is why I suggested that we need to be clear about where the business manager can add value to the new agenda. A business manager should be an analyst of both the internal and external environment and be an agent for change.

Derek Cullen: Individual performance review is probably one of the main fears of consultants about directorates. One can see how one might assess the clinical director or the business manager: if they keep in budget or meet the needs of the community then they get a high grading. However, an individual consultant's role is varied: it varies throughout a professional career from research to clinical work, education, and now management, and many people carry all these things forward at the same time. Am I being naive in thinking that all this will be difficult to assess, or are there methods waiting in the wings to enable consultants to be assessed in the near future?

Cyril Chantler: When you talk about individual performance review,[11] it is important to try to separate the area of staff development from the system of reward, even though you may wish to bring them together again. All who work in an organisation should be aware of that organisation's aims, know the aims of their particular parts in the organisation and how their personal objectives contribute to this. I do not see why they should not discuss these issues on a yearly basis with someone to whom they are managerially accountable within the organisation. Appraisal is a two-way process whereby I, for example, as the principal of a medical school, set out the objectives of the medical school. I also set out my personal objectives, and they are discussed with the chairman of the council of governors. That process is the same throughout the school. I do not see why you cannot have a similar process for consultants in the National Health Service. This is perhaps not so much an appraisal system as a way of making sure that the orchestra plays in tune.

We may be entering a performance related pay system. I have grave doubts about ut whether such a system, as used in some industries, is applicable to the activities of professional staff, be they lawyers, teachers, doctors or nurses. In many industries performance related pay is about motivation. There is plenty of self motivation in the health professions, and there are ways of motivating professional staff other than adding another 10–20% to their pay.

However, I suggest that merit probably needs to be more widely and more openly judged than it is in the present distinction awards system.

Bryan Moore-Smith: The practical problem is that the budget for any salary increment is held centrally and not at directorate level. If that money were devolved to directorates, performance review and reward would be much easier.

Stephen Griffin: I think performance related pay is certainly not the way of the future. It has been discredited in a number of organisations. Applying it in a clinical context is extremely difficult, and even in a managerial context we are about to give our senior managers at St James's notice that we are no longer carrying on with the current arrangements. The issues have to do with who contributes to the success of achieving objectives; many people are involved, not just a few individuals.

Another point to be made is of how one manages employer-wide or hospital-wide strategy, and balances this with the needs of clinical directorates to do their own thing. There are issues such as equal pay for equal work of equal value, and the requirements of legislation. Differences in employment practices in different directorates could generate difficulties for the organisation as a whole. We are still regarded as a trust, as one statutory employer.

Ian Williams: The change that has arisen is that, while clinicians are great self motivators, they motivate themselves to fulfil their own objectives, but are increasingly asked to meet the objectives of an external agency. Maybe one does need to give more thought to how to persuade very motivated people to achieve other people's objectives.

Martin Rossor: To whom should business managers look for their performance review and for their future career advancement? If it is to the centre, how does that affect potentially their loyalty as champion for the directorate?

Andrew Frank: The answer relates in part to the size of the directorate. I am the director of a largish directorate with a budget of £4.5 million, so I hired my business manager. Regrettably I had to fire one. I do not believe my current business manager would doubt that her loyalties are to the clinical directorate.

Wendy Darby: In our hospital our performance review is carried out by the clinical director. He appointed me and therefore he should be reviewing my performance.

Jenny Stephany: There is an issue about who appraises the business manager. At St Mary's the method probably reflects the current centre–directorate tension: it is carried out by the chief executive, the director of operations and the clinical director every six months. This is a fairly tall order because there are many things that the business manager can try to achieve, but most of what a business manager does is achieved through people.

Roger Williams: Where business managers go in terms of promotion is important. We have not had much of this so far because they have all been getting into the job and most of them have been enjoying it. We need to consider soon how best to develop the careers of business managers and their training needs.

John Collinson: There is not yet a specific national training scheme but a two-day conference for business managers will shortly be held at Harrogate.

6 | Management of nursing services within clinical directorates

Martin Severs *General Manager, Elderly Services (Acute)*
Helen Bowers *Elderly Services Manager*
Queen Alexandra Hospital, Cosham, Portsmouth

Nurses are the most numerous and, collectively, the most expensive group of staff in the NHS. Constructive, continuing dialogue between nurses and managers is therefore indispensable for a successful service. Free, open and honest discussion is vital in a clinical directorate; this can be transformed into success when there is a right to be listened to and a commitment to listen. Patient outcomes should be the driving force of the service.

Establishing the clinical directorate

In discussing nurse management within a clinical directorate, it is necessary to look at the organisation itself in terms of both its internal and its external relationships. Three basic models are generally used: the consultant manager, the consultant coordinator and the clinical general manager (see pages 33–35). The structure and shape of directorates are continually changing. The main areas of development surround the practical challenges faced by the common triumvirate version of a clinical directorate, in which the director is supported by a staff manager and a business manager. These challenges include: the practicalities of separating 'staff management' from the management of costs, budgets and business planning; the skill mix of the three people in the triumvirate; and the reliance upon good communication and close relationships for success. Further challenges involve the size and the scope of the clinical directorates and whether, in a large department, the job can be undertaken by a part-time clinician. Variation between clinical directorates affects *who* tackles nursing issues and *how* they do it, but not necessarily *what* issues need tackling.

The main role of consultants within clinical directorates is to understand the purpose and function of the unit and department in which they work. In particular they need a firm grasp of the organisation and functioning of nursing services on a strategic, operational and professional level. Although some nurses have negative attitudes towards clinical directors, it is clear that there are positive benefits for senior nurse managers within clinical directorates. Part of this process may be a natural extension of the clinical partnership the professions have in caring for people.

The second task for consultants within a clinical directorate is to understand their own roles and whether they have the necessary skills and knowledge. This has particular relevance for nursing services. It is helpful to distinguish between strategic, operational and professional issues. The literature concentrates on professional issues and often describes them in emotive language clouded by historical events, such as the debate about the grading of nurses. Such a debate may obscure the boundaries of strategic and operational management, and as a result managers and clinicians may lose sight of the goal of the service—improved patient outcome. Fortunately nurses and other professionals work together in 'real life'; if the organisation is clear about its structure and function, and if the clinical director is explicit about his or her role within it, there are few problems at this stage.

Once the clinical directorate has been established, a number of major strategic, operational and professional issues require attention. Some of them will be peculiar to a locality or specialty, eg in our case the increasing elderly population along the South Coast, but many are generic. An example of the latter is the potential impact of the paper 'Caring for people' on hospital and community services.

Service aims

The most immediate task for a clinical director is to ensure the development of an agreed service philosophy and strategy. This can be derived through a wide variety of formal and informal means but must be patient-focused, developed by all staff within the clinical directorate, and written in a language that can be understood. Unless the nursing staff understand, contribute to and agree with the direction of the service, major problems will arise. These problems stem from a conflict between the perceived management culture of 'business' and the human priorities of nursing. However, anyone who has been through the process of developing a patient-centred strategy quickly learns that apparently large gulfs in cultures may in practice be insignificant.

The service strategy is the foundation for business planning, for quality assurance, and for outcomes management.

Skill mix and workload

Nurses, like many other NHS professionals, are dedicated people who 'through it all grit their teeth and carry on, trying to prove to the world, each other and themselves that they can 'cope' '.[12] This has been encapsulated in Item 11 of the 1984 UKCC Code of Conduct, which stipulated that one should 'have regard to the workload of and the pressure on professional colleagues and subordinates'.[13]

Skill mix is a recurrent theme in any clinical directorate; consultants must understand the principles and the debate over nursing workload and how it should be measured.

Methods for measuring nursing workload are not new or few in number.[14-16] The search for accurate methods to calculate the demand and hence the cost of these services has taken a significant leap up the priority list following the introduction of resource management and the NHS reforms. More than £4.6 billion (almost a quarter of the NHS budget) is spent on nursing each year, and more than half of all health service workers are employed as nurses, so it is easy to see why this area attracts such intense interest. At present 23 nurse management systems are available. They may be dependency driven, 'task' orientated, demand led or, like a minority, may concentrate on care planning. A recent study commissioned by the Department of Health examined the methodologies and assessed the sensitivity and consistency of workload measures.[16]

It is necessary to understand the assumptions and calculations used within a system and the extent to which activity analysis is carried out ward by ward, since all systems ultimately rely on these data and on the method for allocating patients to a particular category. Significant differences in workload have been found when different systems of measurement have been implemented on the same ward, sometimes up to £120,000 per annum. This has led to a major debate over the concept of measurement of workload.

Current measurements of workload cannot cope with the quality with which that work is undertaken, a point worth considering as there does appear to be a definite relation between quality of care and the number of trained nurses on the ward. A simple example is that a decrease in the proportion of trained to untrained staff leads to dramatic increases in waiting times for specialised attention. There is therefore a need for skill mix analysis at a strategic level within a clinical directorate to balance quantity and quality, and there is also a need for operational and professional skills in this measurement.

A welcome initiative entitled 'Using information in managing the nursing resource'[15] has raised operational and professional awareness and skills in this area.

Human resource management

Another complex issue is the time-consuming area of recruitment and retention of nurses. Human resource management has many local as well as national political elements. A recent review of nursing services in the 1990s has identified three key areas: job satisfaction, making better use of nursing skills, and helping nurses combine work and home.

High wastage rates of up to 15% of nurses are reported in some localities, for example, Inner London, Oxford and East Anglia. This is blamed on increasing workloads and cost containment, leading to reduced morale and job satisfaction. Wastage figures can, however, be viewed positively to determine what makes a successful recruiting and retaining organisation. Some hospitals in the USA have been called 'magnet hospitals' because they can attract and retain nursing staff.[17,18] The style of management and the quality of leadership in these hospitals seems to be very important. All had relative organisational stability, with many senior staff working in the same hospital for more than 10 years. Nurse education also appears to be important in retaining nurses.

Nurses contribute to organisational development through participative management and devolved decision making. This is an important strategic message which clinical directors must grasp and which can be developed at an operational level to suit local needs. All major new development bids in our directorate of elderly services are produced by a task force which involves ward level as well as senior clinical nurses. Nurses have also shaped the strategy (the 'mission statements'), and they are fully involved in the discussions about the service and its future. This involvement happened not because we have a high academic staffing quota but because we have a highly skilled workforce whose opinion is valued.

Recruitment and retention policies have ramifications in all aspects of the service; it is a vital area which requires sound managerial skills. Large directorates need a dedicated personnel manager who can offer expertise and experience in tackling the operational processes of advertising, recruitment, maternity and sick leave, resignations and so on. There is also a need to take into account the combination of work and home. One third of NHS nurses are women who work part-time. Most have family commitments which the clinical directorates should try to facilitate in line with the needs of the service.

Training and education

A consistent theme in many of the papers on nursing and its role in the NHS is that of education and development. This aspect was felt to be so important by staff in our directorate that it has become part of our mission statement. It is also, unfortunately, the main area of strife between managers, and between managers and nurses, because nurses want and need education but resources are not available to meet much of that need. Here we do not mean just financial resources; tight staffing establishments make it difficult for services to operate if nurses are away on courses. Within our directorate approximately 0.75% of the nursing establishment is allocated to study leave. We have a mean loss of 1.0% of our nursing staff on study leave at any one time in a one-year period. This barely extends to the desirable educational activities that nursing staff reasonably demand, and hardly covers the essential activities. It is difficult to measure tangible benefits from education, and the internal creation of money for training is nearly impossible when faced with an annual cash releasing efficiency saving of 1.1 %.

Education does not yet appear to be an important organisational area of debate between the purchasers and providers, nor does it feature prominently in the objectives of the NHS management executive. Shenton and Hamm have written that 'employers pay only lip service to the provision of continuing education and many do not make the opportunities which *do* exist sufficiently well known to their staff'.[19]

Education is important and needs clear direction from within the clinical directorates. Certain educational elements are mandatory. Examples include the post-registration education and practice project for trained nurses (which has significant financial and staffing implications), and education about food hygiene, lifting and manual handling of patients, and the control of substances hazardous to health.

Certain educational elements are also of considerable value to the service, for example health care support worker assessor skills, Project 2000[20] assessor skills and English National Board specialty qualifications.

A wide range of mechanisms is needed to obtain measurable increases in the quality or quantity of care that can be achieved through a given educational process, so that development bids in a purchasing environment can be substantiated. Innovative schemes are needed to create the necessary organisational changes to provider units so that education needs are supported. In a time of limited resources, a mechanism is needed to reward the most needy and/or deserving.

Individual performance review

Although not originally designed for this purpose, individual performance review does give a rational base for these decisions, as well as being an important tool in recognising and developing the skills of individuals. According to a recent Institute of Health Services Management report, there appears to be some division of opinion about its value for nurses.[11] This is probably due to differences in the content of objectives in the individual performance review depending on whether they are initiated managerially or clinically. The former are made up of innovatory (50%), maintenance (40%) and personal development (10%) elements and are dominantly service based. The clinically originated objectives tend to concentrate on clinical knowledge and skills, on relationships with patients, staff and carers, and on communication skills.

The practical difficulties of individual performance review in an organisation that creates new management agenda with alarming frequency should not be underrated.

Research and development

Research and development is concerned with patient services, not with tribal loyalties or nursing freedom. It is expanding within provider units. This is not simply in response to the development of a research and development directorate within the NHS management executive but is an essential response to competition in the internal market and the agenda of integrating primary and secondary health care. Nurses are well placed to participate in research and development, and lead in some aspects of this work. This needs to be recognised in the educational needs and career structure of nurses.

Career development

The career structure of nurses requires consideration in every clinical directorate. Most nurses wish to be involved in direct patient care, and the clinical grading structure makes this possible. There are still some problems, notably the relatively large numbers of G grade nurses compared with the number of posts at H or I grades.* For example, in our directorate we have 22 whole-time equivalent (wte) G grade nurses, only two wte H grade posts and no I grade post at all.

There is a well trodden path for nurses from G grade to H grade (part management posts) and then into general management, but little in the way of a purely clinical path apart from posts in highly selective areas, for example in stoma care, continence and diabetes. Lack of clinical career development is a major source of frustration to many nurses. The clinical director should be mindful of this tension in nursing services and should endeavour to improve upon existing systems by making full use of the opportunities offered by research and development for the integration of primary and secondary care, and the shift towards an emphasis on quality and patient outcomes.

Quality and outcomes

The quality of care can be defined as 'the degree to which patient care services (for individuals and populations) increase the probability of desired patient outcomes and reduce the possibility of undesired patient outcomes, given the current state of knowledge',[21] but the dimensions of a quality service are much wider. The common models used are those proposed by Maxwell[22] and Donabedian.[23] The clinical director should enhance the professional responsibilities of the nursing staff in quality and outcomes, and encourage clinical audit. Guidelines for audit of nursing practice are available, but audit is now increasingly seen to be a multidisciplinary task rather than confined to individual professions.[24]

Conclusion

We have avoided making generalisations as to *who* should manage; this would be inappropriate in an overview on such a highly variable managerial concept as that of clinical director, which is still evolving. The words 'to nurse', and 'to nourish' share a

---

Editor's note: The salary scales and responsibilities of nurses are indicated by letters of the alphabet, H and I being the highest grades.

common root. A clinical director should nourish nursing and thereby improve the strategic, operational and professional elements of the service and improve patient outcomes.

In order to measure service outcomes effectively, one needs to develop a thorough system of measuring outcomes, ie outcomes for patients, and what that means for the organisation. That will have an effect on the way the clinical directorate or division is structured from the outset. If one is not geared to measuring benefits for patients, the way the directorate is structured and the way clinical practice is carried out should be reappraised. The service aims of the directorate should be to deliver the best patient care. Clinical audit is now replacing separate nursing quality assurance and medical audit.

DISCUSSION

John Horsley: During my three years as a clinical director, my greatest problem was understanding and trying to get to grips with the nursing budget. I was fortunate in having a good nurse manager with whom I got on well. Nevertheless, I felt at times that I was being led up the garden path as to exactly what was going on within nursing, and other clinicians have reported the same.

Any large hospital still has a chief nurse or matron but the clinical directorate structure has stripped away a fair degree of power from this chief nurse. Decisions can be made in a clinical directorate for good reasons but then the issue of 'quality' comes up and can be used by the chief nurse to stop you introducing change which may indeed be improving quality.

Roger Williams: Along with the chief nurse you have the Royal College of Nursing too. That is a powerful body which still has influence on quality issues, not through clinical directorates but through the chief nurse.

John Horsley: We have already heard about business managers and the way in which business managers have developed. My great concern was the quality of nurse managers we had supporting us within the clinical directorate, and also the degree of support that nurse managers got from ward sisters.

Helen Bowers: Patient care depends on a multidisciplinary approach, particularly when caring for the elderly. That includes not only nurses but also clinicians, consultants—although I do not manage consultants—and therapy staff. Nursing services take up the largest part of my budget. It is complex, and historical factors make it difficult to understand. Having a service manager who is not orientated towards either management or clinical nursing does help nurses to see that they are only one professional group among many.

Christopher Burns-Cox: In the trust in which I work there is a chief nurse who is there for professional advice only. She is not a manager and she would not call herself a manager, although she does do a lot of managing. The only nursing managers are the ward sister and specialist nurses who have their own tiny managerial patch. The senior nurses are not supposed to be nursing managers, and it has been very difficult in a directorate to work with a senior nurse who has been told that she is not in any way to be a manager. How to write a job description for someone who helps the sisters manage their wards yet not call her a manager is very difficult, and we have had great difficulty in getting a job description and making an appointment.

Cyril Chantler: When you think about how much difficulty we doctors have in trying to understand our role within general management and decentralised management, it is hardly surprising that the nurses are having an equally difficult time, even more so when one considers how for the past 20 years in this country they have been pushed through an entirely functional management system as part of the Salmon structure.* Then suddenly, without anybody actually standing up and saying so, the Salmon structure was dismantled. I can understand how difficult it is for senior nurses to accept their new role or even to understand it, and I also understand how much they will resist change.

The new director of nursing at Guy's describes her passion for managing nursing but not nurses. I had exactly the same experience about skill mixes and dependency and so forth, as Robert Tattersall described (see page 22), and I have no doubt that in a sense I was duped. Nurse managers were paraded before me to demonstrate that the staffing levels in our wards were lower than in any other teaching hospital in the whole world and therefore we could not possibly reduce the levels even further. I now realise that this was nonsense. They were talking about structure, stating that if we do not have so many nurses of such and such a grade the service will fall apart and the quality of care will be poor. What is now

*Editor's note: The Salmon structure was a hierarchical system of nurse management, introduced into the NHS in the early 1970s, and now largely defunct, though the Salmon grades remain (see footnote on page 57).

needed are different ways of experimenting with different skill mixes and determining the effect on outcomes, including patient satisfaction.

Derek Cullen: May I ask Helen Bowers if and how she managed to enhance or extend the role of the nurse?

Helen Bowers: This is a development about which the nursing staff seems very enthusiastic. Since nursing services impinge on other professional groups, an extension of the nurse's role involves either taking something away from the junior doctors or the nurses seeing the junior doctors as dumping something on them. We must therefore consider different aspects of care. Who is the right person to do such and such a task? We have to try to get both groups to work through the problem and devise a solution. For example, in regard to death certification at night on our long-stay wards the extended role of the nurses has made a lot of sense and has worked very well. Furthering that role to include our acute medical wards for the elderly and our rehabilitation wards is still under negotiation because of different aspects of care. Successful negotiation depends on whether the nursing staff see a task as a downgrading of their role—an assistant to the junior doctor rather than a professional in their own right. If the task can be identified as professional and should be carried out by a nurse, there has so far been no problem in implementing the change.

7 | An appropriate career structure for the clinical director

Roger Williams
*Second Vice-President, Royal College of Physicians,
and Director, Institute of Liver Studies,
King's College School of Medicine and Dentistry, London*

A central plank of the government's attempt to improve efficiency in the NHS over the past five years is a greater involvement of hospital consultants in the management process. It has been hoped that clinicians would develop a greater role in all-important decisions relating to clinical priorities and the use of resources. Initial experience with clinical directorates (or 'care groups' as they are sometimes termed) at Guy's Hospital was encouraging and, although there has been no uniform pattern, these are now in place in most of our hospitals. As the NHS reforms began to be introduced, the work of the directorates took on an extra dimension with respect to the content of contracts with purchasing authorities and to a number of quality issues. Consultants at first found that they had not enough administrative and secretarial support, but many directorates now have a business manager, a nurse with experience in management, and others with specific administrative skills within the management team. With budgets properly devolved to the directorates, rationalisation within and between clinical services becomes a possibility. However, some affirm that only the unpleasant tasks have been fully handed over by the chief executive and trust board and that there is an even tighter bureaucratic control from central management. Indeed in some hospitals consultants have become disenchanted with the process and have been replaced by non-medical managers of directorates.

Part of the disenchantment almost certainly relates to the rapidly increasing extent and complexity of the work involved; as the effects of the NHS reforms are beginning to be seen, there is no likelihood that managerial needs will lessen. The one or two sessions that were given over to clinical directorate work seem to have extended to three or four. Conflicts with clinical work are an inevitable result, especially for those in teaching hospitals with the additional requirements of academic activity and research. However, as clinical directorates are more effectively constructed, it should be possible to define what is really required of the clinical directors, so that they can maintain their clinical experience on which their value in the management team at least partly depends.

Administrators receive performance bonuses, and the doctor's contribution in the clinical directorate must similarly be adequately recompensed. Some way of giving recognition to the importance of such posts in the medical staff structure also needs to be found. The way consultant work was established in the NHS leads to difficulties in setting up a more hierarchical system to encompass the wider role and greater responsibilities of the clinical director. There are current discussions about the wider introduction of the specialist grade. These doctors will have acquired a certain level of professional knowledge but not yet become consultants. Promotion to the consultant grade would depend upon additional responsibilities in patient care and organisational work within the hospital. For each category of appointment (hospital specialist, consultant, clinical director) there needs to be a separate salary scale, with an allowance for seniority. The doctor appointed to a post as clinical director will have to acquire extra knowledge and skills in health service organisation, in management accountancy and in information technology, so that he or she is as expert and informed in these new areas of work as in clinical practice. Attendance at instructional and interactive courses is likely to be part of this and will need facilitating (see Chapter 8).

There is increasing pressure from purchasing authorities and general practitioner fundholders for clinical work in hospitals to become more consultant based. It follows that only with a considerable increase in consultant numbers will it be possible to do this, as well as to accommodate the extra workload resulting from the managerial responsibility of clinical directorates. When new consultant posts are funded they will need to be allocated to the medical specialties from which clinical directors are so often drawn, as well as to the areas of present apparent shortage.

We also need to consider how, as clinical director, one can influence the quality of practice of other doctors. One of the most difficult parts of being a clinical director is to influence your consultant colleagues since they do not always agree with you! The person selected for such a post must have considerable credibility as a leader in his or her own clinical specialty or in some field of medicine, and also personal credibility. There is obvious benefit in the appointment of directors who have the full support of their colleagues; the choice should not be made purely on the basis of seniority or status but it would be difficult for a registrar or senior registrar suddenly to be put in charge of a clinical directorate. In practice, choice is frequently determined by the lack of interested or suitable candidates.[25,26] There are not many consultants who want to come forward for these positions. Where the clinical directorate scheme has been a success, consultants are keen to become clinical directors; where it is not a success there is a general disillusionment and difficulty in filling clinical director posts.

Consultants were primarily trained as clinicians and remain individualists. Often they do continue with the same clinical workload and do not give up anything when they take on the extra responsibilities of a clinical director. Consultants may sometimes have difficulty in becoming part of a team, even the leader of a team, because they usually think they know what is best. Berwick has written: 'They arrive late or not at all at meetings. They dominate when they are present. They sometimes leap to solutions before the team has done its proper diagnostic work on the process. They do with processes what they would rarely do with patients—assume that they have the answer even before the question has been clearly formulated or the data have been collected.'[27]

There are potential tensions in the relationship between clinical directors and the chief executive of a trust. There has to be a proper delegation of both budget and responsibility to the clinical director. But relinquishing power is not easy. Some chief executives use the clinical directors to do some of their dirty work, ie work that they have never been able to do themselves and which they now believe they will be able to do by having consultants in that role.

At the same time, clinical directors have not to be sucked so far into the management process that they lose contact or involvement in clinical work which would diminish credibility as a clinical director. Clinical directors also have to be particularly careful about seeking personal or professional advantages by virtue of their position in the hierarchy. If unwise about this, there will be trouble with the other consultants in the clinical directorate. It is a recipe for disaster if consultant leaders are seen to gain, either in terms of what they can do for their patients or in other ways, by virtue of their position in management.

I list below what I consider necessary for success as a clinical director:

• Proper delegation of authority from the chief executive, and at the same time proper involvement in the overall affairs of the hospital

- Adequate support from other staff (business manager, senior nurse, personnel department, etc)
- Proper balance between management role (three to four sessions) and clinical responsibilities (six to seven sessions)
- Sufficient training in, for example, organisation of services, management, accountancy, information technology
- Proper recognition of role and work in terms of remuneration and career structure

The first requirement is proper authority. At King's College Hospital we started with an involvement at senior level in a clinical board. All the clinical directors were part of the clinical board, which in turn related closely to the chief executive. But the chief executive has appointed non-medical administrators at a managerial level above all the clinical directors, who now feel that their involvement in the affairs of the hospital is at best third-hand. It seems that there has not been sufficient trust in the clinical directors and their ability to perform the role desired of them; it may be that they have not performed well enough. Along with the change in the system, so few recruits are coming forward to take these positions that at least half of the eight or nine clinical directorates are now directed by non-medical, non-consultant people.

The next need is for adequate support staff. The business manager, the senior nurse and the personnel function are all crucial. The third need is for enough time. Cyril Chantler said it would be possible to act effectively as clinical director in one or two sessions. That is probably true, although I would set a slightly different balance between management and clinical responsibilities. It is possible to do more clinical work if the support structure is in place, and if proper loyalties develop so that you are not worried about the business manager spending all his or her time in the chief executive's office and not looking after your care group or clinical directorate's work.

We also have to consider what happens to former clinical directors. Clinical directors who enjoy their work and have been successful should be able to go into higher levels of management in the hospital. The sort of career structure that I have outlined, with separate salary levels for each of the grades, would recognise the role of the clinical director and how that evolves in terms of one's professional life and training. Indeed, unless some such scheme is put in place, we will never really establish this clinical director role for consultants.

8 | What are the skills required and training needs of clinical directors?

Judith Riley
Fellow in Management Education,
King's Fund College, London

Several generalised descriptions of the job of clinical director are available, as well as hundreds of individual job specifications. For example, the Middlesex Business School used one (see Appendix 1 page 97) as part of an evaluation of the NHS management executive funded initiative, which has paid for more than 300 consultants to attend business schools and join learning sets.[28] It asks questions about 38 key tasks, divided into groups as follows:

> 4 about relationships with colleagues
> 2 about policy and strategy
> 6 about budgeting
> 11 about managing people
> 5 about managing change
> 3 about managing information
> 7 about personal competencies

Wraith Casey management consultants produced another example, in the form of a checklist for self-appraisal or reviewing performance (see Appendix 2 page 99).[26] They based this on looking at the emergence of clinically based management at the Wirral Hospital Trust. Their questions were grouped as follows:

> 13 about overall management practice
> 9 about teamwork
> 2 about communication
> 8 about decision making
> 10 about leadership style
> 12 about culture and climate

Another set of priorities emerged from a recent conference on managing clinical services—decentralisation in action. We asked a group of about 40 doctors to do some rapid brainstorming around their worries and say what they considered were the key factors for success as clinical directors. The full list is in Appendix 3 (page 102). The main issues that concerned them were:

- Directorate structures: what is the ideal number of directorates and how should their heads be related to managers?
- How does the director role fit into a clinical career, how should it be remunerated, and how should clinical cover be provided?
- What training and support are needed to do the job?

Training available

Training for such tasks and abilities is increasingly available, through regional health authority training centres, several universities and within individual hospitals. The Open University courses for health professionals and their basic, more general management courses offer what is essentially high quality education by correspondence. The King's Fund offers a variety of courses, including a basic 5-day programme for inexperienced clinical directors; other centres provide shorter courses or a series of seminars. The five days of our own course are divided up roughly into one and a half hour sessions:

- Introductions and exploring participants' agenda
- Management issues for the 1990s
- Where is the NHS going?
- Why should consultants bother about management?
- Finance and budgets (two sessions)
- Personal reflections on being a clinical and medical director
- Improving quality and the role of audit (two sessions)
- Contractual relationships (three sessions)
- Managing clinical work through contracts (two sessions)
- Personal development: careers, time priorities and self-presentation (three sessions)
- Options of the clinicians' choosing, usually management skills such as negotiation or managing people (four sessions)

One of the obvious problems with such training is that owing to the limited time available there must be very selective or superficial cover of each essential skill or area of knowledge. Two or three hours on dealing with financial information is always appreciated, but it is difficult to progress from learning about it to learning to do it, making the skill directly usable at work. A business manager may prepare budgets, but the clinical director needs to be able to check them and discuss them. Interactive courses that encourage discussion and use a workshop approach with simulations, questionnaires and role-playing are likely to be more effective than courses of lectures alone.

Even inexperienced clinical directors have individual profiles of development needs: they all have different strengths and weaknesses. Specially designed sessions to meet the most pressing needs of the participants provide one answer. Small group options also allow some individualisation of a programme. Access to a wide range of books and videos, with time for individual study, represents a third approach.

Deeper dilemmas

Although a well designed course or workshop can be helpful, some clinical directors have experienced and valued a deeper level of training. A small group of participants at one of our courses recently reported that these attempts to identify tasks or required skills and to train in them were only the first stage. It had helped them to see such job descriptions, to learn about management and to develop their management skills, but they had also needed more. One of them said 'You *want* that kind of training but you *need* something else'.

I have found that, when clinical directors are with others, they trust each other and feel safe enough to voice their real fears and worries. A new level of questions then emerges; for example, they ask each other about the following areas.

Dealing with difficult colleagues

How can the clinical director deal with a difficult colleague, such as a bright young consultant who is improving standards without paying attention to the stress caused to the nurses? The concept of working in a multidisciplinary and mutually dependent team is accepted by the clinical director but foreign to this new colleague.

Alternatively, the problem may be an older consultant who will not consider the evidence that his or her practice needs to change, is always too busy to attend clinical audit meetings and does not realise that the referral load is increasing for his or her colleagues. The culture of openness and peer review for continuous improvement is not accepted by everyone.

The difficult person might be a manager who will not let the director meet those who purchase directorate services. Such a manager has not understood that decentralised clinical management is not just about dumping financial accountability on doctors; rather it is essential to involve clinicians in contracting, if the highest feasible quality of care is to be achieved.

Relationships with colleagues

Are relationships going to change? Does the clinical director
inevitably become to some degree identified with management
who may be seen as the enemy? Does the director risk being treated as a traitor? Must long-term working friendships suffer as the
director distances himself or herself from particular cronies, or
colleagues find themselves covering some of the director's work
with no apparent special benefit to their department?

How selfish may one be?

What is the real aim of accepting a clinical director job? Is there a
hidden agenda? Some clinical directors say that a few directors in
their hospital use their new post to help their own small department. More experienced directors see emerging dilemmas in balancing their concern for their own hospital with that for all hospitals in the area. Yet others see the dilemmas in terms of my
patients, our patients, all patients, or all potential patients. Short-
term or long-term planning can produce yet another tension.

To lead or to follow

Directors begin to see that different areas of their hospital or community service are in different positions along the path of transi-
tion from the old world to the new. Some parts are still thinking in
old style block funding terms, while others have switched to the
new style culture of funding by contracts. Some consultants still
assume job security, while others know that their jobs depend on
their ability to attract paid work. Some still believe they are in control of rationing through their waiting lists; others realise that this
problem has now passed to their purchasers. Some still insist on
doing whatever tests and treatments they judge to be best, while
others have accepted professional accountability for the use of
resources.

The dilemma is how to position oneself as a clinical director in
relation to one's colleagues, the management board and the purchasers of the services provided by the directorate. Most clinical
directors want to lead, but stepping too far ahead can daunt one's
colleagues. Trying to lead without strong management support for
a clinical director's efforts is impossibly frustrating and time-consuming.

Career planning

For many consultants, the move into a clinical director post may signal the first time that they have to make difficult career choices. They have so far been moving up a single ladder and now find that the ladder has branches. How far do they want to move towards management, which can appear not only exciting and important but also daunting and frustrating? Might they want a medical director role next, or eventually want to be chief executive of a trust?

Another fundamental dilemma is about the future of the clinical director role. There is an assumption that clinical directors are a good thing and here to stay. Some directors question this in private and wonder whether they may not be able to achieve more for their hospital by pursuing the traditional routes to influence, such as chairing the medical staff committee.

Helping with the deeper dilemmas

Many new clinical directors want to look at job descriptions and questions that allow them to assess their own performance, and they feel more comfortable when they have had some essential skills and knowledge training. Then they find that they are facing deeper dilemmas, such as those outlined above, which involve their attitudes and values. Conventional management courses and books are unlikely to be of much help. However, three forms of further development have been rated as valuable.

Experience exchange

Clinical directors from different areas of the country seem to have an enormous amount to offer each other. The very differences in their circumstances show new ways of interpreting the role, new possibilities for relationships, and new ways of tackling the really difficult problems.

Small 'learning sets' of four to six clinical directors meeting for a couple of days every two to three months can soon be helped to trust each other and to find their own agenda and ways of working. They do need sensitive leadership to help the group to get on well and to feel safe enough to tackle what is personally difficult. Selection is also necessary to ensure a wide range of experience and avoid potential problems relating to confidentiality.

One important insight gained by these groups is that there are no neat answers out there or in the textbooks. Hospitals and community services may sometimes seem nearly unmanageable. It is easy for directors and managers to feel responsible for all their problems. Directing clinical colleagues has been likened to 'herding cats'. The search for the best solution, and the hard data to support it, can be the enemy of the 'good enough' answer which can at least be implemented.

Personal development

By personal development I mean becoming more aware of one's own strengths and weaknesses and of how others react to one's behaviour. It means becoming able to hear and observe nuances, to drop old and now inappropriate behaviours, to bring more of oneself to work, dropping many unnecessary defences. Clinical directors are no longer learning about something but rather are changing in themselves, becoming happier, more confident and more able to listen and learn and to ask for help. Personal development of this kind appears to be very welcome to many clinical directors and may be helped by feedback organised by skilled facilitators.

Manager allies

My colleagues and I are now often called to help with directorate 'away days', where the ostensible agenda of reviewing services and developing business plans is generally agreed to be less important than enabling clinicians and managers to work together. The discovery that former enemies are allies under the skin can be disconcerting; finding mutual respect for each other's skills and knowledge can be both exciting and comforting.

There is a growing demand for learning sets which include both managers and clinical directors and a few other key professionals. For example, five members in one of my sets had experience in the following posts:

- Director of clinical services
- Clinical director, with experience of various multidisciplinary quality initiatives
- Community unit general manager, formerly a nurse
- Unit general manager of a hospital about to become a trust
- Chief executive of a large group of acute hospitals, formerly a district general manager.

Another set brought together the following:

- Medical adviser for acute services to a large purchasing authority, formerly a medical director
- Chief executive of a district general hospital, formerly a clinician

- Assistant regional general manager, formerly a worker in local government
- Director of purchasing, formerly a planner
- Director of personnel for a teaching hospital, formerly NHS management executive and civil servant in a government department other than health

In such mixed groups, clinical directors both find fresh perspectives and obtain inside knowledge of other key professions.

Conclusions

It may help to think of training for the role of clinical director as being at two levels. The first level is management training for a particular setting and builds confidence. It is similar to the training needed by the nurse manager or business manager. However, clinical directors usually have other deeper dilemmas, which cannot be significantly helped by this first level of training. Various forms of exchanging experience, multiprofessional teamwork and personal development offer more and may be seen as a second level of training, which requires time and funding in its own right.

In accepting the onerous position of clinical director, I believe one should negotiate for time and money to be put aside for second level training, as well as the more obvious first level.

The first question asks where the money comes from and where the time comes from. The second question is whether such deeper training should be undertaken within individual hospitals or arranged across hospitals; is it done with just other clinical and medical directors, or is it done with other professionals and managers in the health service and, perhaps, even outside the NHS, for example with colleagues in social services or from the private health care industry or the voluntary sector?

DISCUSSION (Chapters 7 and 8)

Robert Tattersall: Roger Williams suggested that expert doctors might progress to higher levels of management and move away from hands-on care. We must not have a final arrow, leading irrevocably to management alone.

Roger Williams: Some doctors who have shown their skills as clinical director may want to go on to a career more orientated towards general management, or become an NHS trust chief executive. I was trying to convey the point that, if clinical directors are to do their jobs properly for three to five years and have some position with respect to their consultant colleagues, consultants cannot all be on the same level. This is one of the problems. Every consultant in the NHS is on the same basic contract. You do get additional contracts giving perhaps one or two sessions as clinical director, but still you are regarded by everybody as a consultant. It is necessary to recognise that there are elements of a hierarchical system here.

Eve Wiltshaw: I agree with Roger Williams that you should have some kind of hierarchical system for clinical management, but I would like to see a tree, not a ladder. One of the major problems of medical staffing is the expectation that a doctor who gets into hospital and stays two or three years will inevitably become a consultant, or fail. This is nonsense; no other career progression ever implies that you start off with 100 people and end up with 100 people at the top. We ought to have levels at which people will wish to stop, and we ought to encourage people to move both up and down.

David Walker: Everyone has a right to personal development and growth. Yorkshire regional health authority runs a management training scheme which has given opportunities for doctors to take part in consultancy and counselling programmes along with managers. Development of skills has been multidisciplinary and has brought together members of the service who, to a certain extent, have not shared their experience in the past.

Wendy Darby: It is important to think about the clinical service team as a whole and not just consider the role of the clinical director. You can then help to break down some of the barriers, share some of the responsibility and develop all-important trust.

A trust board needs to consider what contracts to offer the nurse manager, the business manager and the clinical director. A contract should not automatically move from one consultant to another; if the successor is not experienced or does not have the appropriate management skills, three or four years' of good work may quickly be lost. Future clinical directors ought to be trained now, not suddenly when they are appointed. It is also important that the whole hospital should have some form of induction training programme for the clinical service team as a whole, so that if there is a change of personnel the newly appointed person will be rapidly trained in order that everybody has the same level of understanding of how teams and directorates operate.

Andrew Franks: One problem is that information about many of the programmes for training and development is circulated two to four months previously to those who might be interested. This is inappropriate for people with major clinical responsibilities whose patient waiting lists may extend up to six months. It is not so easy to cancel clinics, particularly if you provide a service that may be individualistic or specialised and where there is no one who automatically steps into your shoes. The NHS management executive should plan courses on a regular basis, so that it is possible to plan 6–12 months ahead what your management needs might be or what your potential successor's management needs might be.

In ceasing to be a clinical director there should be no loss of face. Clinicians should have opportunities for returning to clinical work, at a senior and advisory level. Furthermore, not everybody will want to become a medical director, even if the opportunities are there. It is important to provide opportunities for service development when young consultants have energies for that, and not to postpone the opportunities until just before retirement.

Eve Wiltshaw: The skills and strengths mentioned in Chapter 7, if fulfilled, would fit a doctor to run a corporation! I do not think we can expect clinical directors, who really are fairly lowly managers, to have all those abilities.

Doctors may not realise that they have been managers all their lives. They manage their patients, they manage their junior staff, and some manage laboratories and laboratory staff. The problem we face is our peers: we do not hire and we do not fire consultants; we do not have appropriate sticks or carrots—any good things to offer to collaborative and helpful consultants. We need to explore how to cope with the few colleagues who do not cooperate in the smooth running of the directorate and in the appropriate provision of services to patients.

Judith Riley: I agree that an early part of the training of clinical directors is to convince consultants that they already are managers and have an enormous amount of managerial experience. I also agree that anyone who had all the skills I outlined could run a corporation. The job description for a clinical director is crazy; nobody could do all that in half a day a week or one day a week, or even two days a week.

I think that my chapter and the appendices reveal something of the job of a clinical director and how wide-ranging it is. Crucial for success must be the skills of the business manager and the nurse manager, and trust in their skills. If they are good enough, and if they really work for the clinical director rather than for central management, and if the clinical director can trust them and work together as a team, clinical directors need little training beyond their existing consultant management experience.

Helen Bowers: Training for the business or service manager is important, so that their knowledge parallels that gained by the clinical director. This can be achieved by offering training opportunities for young or junior managers to learn about clinical and service issues while they are learning to be managers; in that way you have the best of both worlds.

Robert Tattersall: We continue to be divided about how much time the work of a clinical director requires. When I first took on the job in our hospital, my manager said that I could do it in one session. I wrote my own job description, and I reckoned that it would take between four and five sessions a week, a time similar to that suggested by Roger Williams. Either I need to go on a course in time management or the job really does take this amount of time. Once the directorate has been set up and is running, that time could probably be reduced, but I do not think it will ever be less than about three sessions a week, even though I have a nurse manager and a business manager on whom I can rely.

Martin Severs: It depends on the size of the organisation you are managing and the number of support staff you have. I have found it relatively easy to run a clinical directorate with a budget of £3 million and 250 employees. Now that I have a budget of about £7.5 million and 550 employees, I need to commit a lot of time, including evenings and weekends, even though I have a good team.

Jenny Stephany: The critical factors relate to what tasks the clinical director thinks only he or she can do, and what tasks can be and are delegated. The directorate must have channels of communication to ascertain who is doing what, to ensure that complementary rather than duplicated work takes place.

Andrew Frank: Another issue is the pace of change. You cannot continue with a limited management team and budget and limited time if you are to develop. For example, if the clinical director is planning or setting up a new discharge scheme of considerable proportions, or winding down some activity, more time is required. Furthermore, purchasers may demand movement in some areas and not in others. It is important, therefore, not to have fixed guidelines as to what is right and what is not right in terms of time and support. The chief executive needs flexibility in order to support the directorates that are clearly moving.

Stephen Griffin: I spend four or five sessions a week, and additional time at home, on managing my directorate, and I have very good support. If you are trying innovative systems of care, or planning a new medical block, or trying to integrate acute and elderly medicine, or dealing with junior doctors' hours and so on, you have to do many of these things yourself or be personally involved in them, just to carry credibility with your colleagues. If you just hand everything on to a business manager and tell him or her to come back in two days with the answer, you will lose credibility. You really have to do a lot of the work yourself.

In addition you will find that the central management structure of the hospital also needs your skills. If you are doing a good job as clinical director, the chief executive will quickly realise that and want your help with other problems within the hospital. So, if you are not careful you will be asked to do a great many extra things. This is why people complain about lots of extra meetings. But there is no doubt that if you work as a clinical director in a large district hospital covering acute and elderly medicine, with 300–400 beds and 600–700 staff and a budget of £5–10 million, no matter how good your business manager is (and anyway you do not know how long your business manager is going to stay with you), you are involved in a lot of hard work. People who say you do not need much time make me wonder what is going on in their organisations.

Eve Wiltshaw: I agree with what has been said about the pace of change, and it does not look as though the pace will let up for some time. I started with four sessions as clinical director, and dropped part of my clinical practice. I then kept a diary which showed that I was doing 18 hours a week in addition to the four session. Now I am doing, theoretically, six sessions. I am paid for six sessions but do eight, and still there are not enough hours in the day. Keeping in touch with consultants, and maintaining the flow of information and discussion, takes a long time, not through hundreds of meetings but in responding to colleagues who otherwise become unhappy. I do not see why doctors should be able to manage in a short space of time and do it well when the posts of chief executive, business manager and nurse are all full-time; why can they not do in three sessions what we are expected to do?

Christopher Burns-Cox: It is necessary to strike a balance between a 'centrifugal' and a 'centripetal' clinical director. When there is a problem, I consider first whether it can be satisfactorily delegated. In order to function one has to remain sane, so delegation is my first priority.

Next, it is of enormous help to have the offices of the directorate in the right position. If you have an office next to your manager, you are more likely to meet in the corridor, or you can just drop in and solve a problem over a cup of coffee. You also need considerable support from a personal assistant or secretary. The secretary who services me and the business manager is the key person: she keeps the diary, organises us all, and removes a lot of the hassle.

Andrew Frank: We have not yet discussed the management of space; this is crucial in any organisation since output depends upon the efficient utilisation of space which is now subject to capital charges. Clinical directors need to consider these costs in their contracting and in planning future developments.

Anthony Hopkins: Possession of space is power. Formerly it was possession of beds, but this no longer cuts much ice. The people who have the most power in an institution are those who control the space and also who can call the most meetings.

Robert Tattersall: The amount of time you spend depends on how much you decide to do. After I had resigned as clinical director I began to think the problem was that I had tried to be all things to all people, but one of the best things I had done was to attend the ward sisters' monthly meeting and a three-monthly meeting for ward receptionists. The morale of the receptionists was unbelievably improved because, they said, no one in management had ever appeared to be interested in them before. So, with quite simple measures, although they take time, you can greatly improve morale and probably the directorate's function.

Jenny Stephany: It seems that the major contribution a clinical director can make is to identify the key issues. Although there is a great need for all kinds of discussion and communication, it is more important to concentrate on a few key issues than to work 23 or 24 hours a day. There are perhaps ten issues that are important within a directorate at any time, and the director should focus on them.

Anthony Hopkins: Has anyone here had to ask a consultant colleague in the directorate to stop doing something that is inappropriate, ineffective or unnecessary, such as admitting patients for an investigation that could be carried out in the outpatient department and may not even be appropriate? Were they successful, and how did they achieve this?

Roger Williams: People have had very little success in influencing clinical practices of other consultants within their clinical directorates. I would be surprised if people here can quote specific instances in which they succeeded.

Bryan Moore-Smith: I have certainly seen a change in practice, for example a willingness to spend more time training junior staff, simply because of unspoken peer pressures. You have to take a medium to long-term view. If you think you will change the world or an individual by Wednesday, you are probably wrong. If the same problem turns up each month in the budget statement, and colleagues start saying 'You are spending £2000 a month more than I am: what is the benefit to your patient?', the message starts to get home and people do respond. It does not happen overnight but it does happen over a period of time, and fairly painlessly.

Martin Rossor: An example of professional practice and the use of resources in my specialty of neurology concerns imaging. Resource consumption seems to depend on who holds the budget: if colleagues have to pay for those CT scans, they stop doing them, but if I have to pay for them, they take no notice of me whatsoever!

Ian Williams: There are instances where you can get much more rapid change. For example, we managed to use our beds more efficiently when we introduced a programmed investigation unit for specific investigations. Colleagues indicated that they would not use the facility but, once they realised that it gave them more beds to do other things they wanted to do, we achieved much higher throughput.

We also looked at drug expenditure in the intensive care unit. Again it became apparent that one or two consultants were behaving differently from others. We were assured that the differences were accounted for by case mix, but fortunately, because the numbers were few, we could analyse patient management in some detail. Case mix did not account for that different practice of our colleagues. For example, some treated status epilepticus with intravenous sodium valproate which is nine times as expensive as the equally effective phenytoin. Our colleagues have now changed their practice.

Eve Wiltshaw: Most people are easily persuaded by facts. As far as drugs are concerned, we help change through a drugs and therapeutics committee which gives guidelines, but any consultant who continually abuses them is asked to come to the committee and explain. Consultants have their peers around the table and they have to argue why they continue such and such a practice, and often are unable to support their previous actions. If someone is very difficult, there is no reason why one should not have a kind of informal disciplinary action group. This could consist, for example, of the director of clinical services, the operational services director and the personnel director. There does come a time when you have to take the bit between your teeth, but you must be sure to have the support of your chief executive and most of your colleagues.

John Horsley: Is one way forward through clinical audit in the directorate? One ploy is simply to get the person who you know to be using an unusual method of treatment to be the chairperson for that particular audit, and to undertake, with any necessary help, the background research before the audit meeting.

Anthony Hopkins: Audit, which certainly should be based within the clinical directorate, is useful for encouraging the recognition of variations in length of stay and use of drugs. What is more difficult is the hope of the Department of Health that outcomes of care will be auditable. There are certainly some adverse outcomes that are auditable, but case mix often makes it difficult to discover whether one doctor is clinically as effective as another.[29,30]

Jenny Stephany: In our directorate we do, on many occasions, send problems for solution down the 'audit channel' rather than the 'business manager channel'.

Roger Williams: Another part of the structure of the directorate to be remembered is the younger doctors in training. Senior registrars are now becoming interested in management and want to go on courses and so on. We should therefore persevere in trying to obtain a good structure for clinical directorates, because there is enthusiasm for them and benefits may come from them.

Judith Riley: A lot of what I have called first level management training is now being given to senior registrars, and is accepted by them as appropriate for the jobs they are doing now as well as the jobs they will do as consultants in the future.

I wonder whether, if this group were to meet again in five or ten years time, many of the members would be senior registrars who would be playing a major management role in relation with business managers and nurse managers. Consultants would be real influences for change, even forces for change, within a hospital, without necessarily being labelled 'clinical director' or 'medical director'. Perhaps it would be back to the chair of the staff committee. Other positions might be much more powerful in the future: I am not at all sure that the structure at present being promoted by Cyril Chantler is the one for ever.

I also think that there would be not only more senior registrars here but also more managers. Chief executives working with clinical directors and directors of medical services constitute a powerful combination for changing a hospital. Managers desperately need to understand your world—the clinical world—far more than they do at present. They need hospital consultants to help them to see how this world can be moved and shifted. There is also a great deal that hospital consultants can learn from managers.

9 | The future of clinical directorates

Robert Maxwell
Chief Executive and Secretary,
King Edward's Hospital Fund for London

I have no doubt about the importance of a strong bond between the professional activity in an institution or agency and its general management. The bond is necessary in all professions that work with and within a larger organisation, for example engineering, much of the law, and the church. In designing buildings and getting them built, or in running an arts organisation or a law firm, there are some elements that are familiar in all: high powered individuals doing something that they have skill in doing and training to do, but which is essentially based upon a dynamic that may be at odds with some of the dynamics of the institution itself. No institution or set of services will work well if the functional and institutional activities are not in balance. In health care this dual function and responsibility is evident from:

- the need for several professions to work together, each exercising professional judgement in its own field;
- the tension between the needs of one patient and the needs of others—a tension that is not well recognised in the Hippocratic tradition;
- the difficulty and pain of some of the decisions that have to be made, in conjunction with patients and their families, about when to treat and when not to do so;
- the tightness of resource constraints and the need for choices within the available resources that clearly ought to be professionally informed, but equally are public policy choices for which the institution is publicly accountable.

Clinical directorates in the form described in this book are one means of achieving such a bond, and that is why they are important. They are not an end in themselves but a means to an end. They are not guaranteed to work; most of all they depend on competent people, committed to leadership roles, and on confidence in the arrangements from both the professional and the general management sides. When they work, the effect can transform an institution, but you cannot necessarily assume that the impact is permanent. Clinical directorates may be more fragile than most people recognise. Once they deteriorate and confidence in them weakens on either the professional or the general management side, they are hard to rebuild.

The only alternative to an effective bond of this kind is to have professionals either working in the institution but not as part of it, or firmly under the general management thumb and doing what they are told. Either of these alternatives is 'bad news'.

There are really only two alternative ways of running a hospital, one at each end of the spectrum. In one you view the hospital or the institution as a series of workshops in which the professionals do their own things in their own way, and what goes on in the institution as a whole is of no concern to them, so long as their workshop gets lighted, warmed and cleaned. That is, in one sense, the traditional view of at least some hospitals. At the other end of the spectrum you get to the position that I have seen in parts of Eastern Europe in the old days, where the senior clinicians did what they were told by clinician-managers even more senior than themselves. I do not think that is a good model either.

I favour the middle of this spectrum and some balance between institutional and clinical interests. We have to find a way for those two to work well together. Clinical directorates are just one way of finding a balance. In my opinion they are to be taken no more seriously than that: they are a way of doing something that has to be done if we are to have effective health care organisations for the future. If clinical directorates do not work, we must find some other mechanism. In any case, there is considerable variation between directorates: at meetings of this kind people using the same terms may mean slightly different things, depending on their own experience.

For example, nursing is an integral part of some clinical directorates and is managed within the directorate. In others nursing is not managed within the directorate but centrally, the directorate having a service agreement with the central nursing organisation as to what nursing services it wants and will pay for. These are two very different models for a clinical directorate. Whenever we talk of specific circumstances, I think we would find substantial differences around the room and around the country.

In organisation there are few scientific certainties and a great deal of fashion. The idea of clinical directorates could go out of fashion; they will certainly become less novel and a part of the established order of things. If they do go out of fashion because they are not seen to be working, we must seek something else, but at present I do not see a better alternative. Clinical directorates must have the confidence and backing of both general management and clinicians. If backing and confidence are lost they will be very difficult to rebuild, and if people have put a lot of effort into trying to make something happen in management it will be more difficult to persuade them to try a second time.

There is a mismatch between authority and responsibility. It is all very well to give people high sounding titles, and it is amazing how some will take on jobs that seem important even if rather thankless. But people in such jobs must have the authority to accompany the responsibility they hold, and I believe such authority has to be negotiated.

A certain amount of authority can and must be given by the institution. For example, clinical directorates must have authority over their own budget within agreed rules. To my mind, this means not only authority over expenditure but also over income. Directorates need to be responsible for negotiating the terms of their contracts and then adjusting their expenditure to match.

Equally, authority has to be negotiated by the clinical directorate with the clinicians, because being a clinical director is to an extent a kind of elected role as well as an appointed role. It is a role that you can fill only if you have the confidence of your colleagues as well as having authority from the institution. Part of the authority from colleagues has to be what colleagues give up to, or give to, the directorate, as long as they have confidence in it; they surrender some things that are precious to them. These may include resource issues, such as how beds or junior staff are assigned, but colleagues will need to have common views on issues relating to quality. Money, important as it is, is not the most important thing in health care but simply a constraint; what is important in health care is the quality and effectiveness of the care given. Unless clinical directorates concern themselves with these, what are they actually up to?

Management is specific to the time and the context in which it has to be carried out. I mean that there is a diagnostic element, the definition of what sort of management or leadership is needed in a particular service or institution at a particular time. Clinical directors must therefore be clear-headed about what they can realistically achieve in the time available, not only in their sessional time but for the duration of their contract. You must ask yourself what things it is important to get done in your time, in your service, in your institution, and focus effort on those. The team of clinical director, business manager, nurse manager and so on must be interdependent to be effective. It must have a clear, shared idea of where its focus lies and what it is trying to do, and how individual roles fit together: who will try to do what? We have not really touched on morale—how people feel about the job they are doing—since that ultimately will make more difference than anything else to the quality of work done, and perhaps even to how the success of the directorate is perceived.

Conclusion

What, then, are the necessary components for a successful directorate structure? As a starting point I suggest:

- The number of directorates needs to be great enough to reflect the real variety of clinical activity (ie the equivalent of strategic business units), but they need to be grouped so that the directorates influence strategy and resource allocation for the whole institution.
- There must be a starting commitment from both the professional side (nursing as much as medicine) and the general management side to make the arrangements work. If either commitment weakens, it must be re-established if directorates are to fulfil their function.
- Directorates must be given as much autonomy as possible for expenditure, income, workload and quality, within strategic parameters agreed by general management.
- Clinical directors must have authority to deal with problems within their directorate, and general management must provide support. The remedy if a clinical director acts irresponsibly is to remove him or her from the post. Of course this is not a sanction to use lightly, and a wise clinical director will not in any case spring surprises on general management about important issues.
- Clinical directorates must meet their targets (see above). A director who fails to do so must be subject to proper discipline and ultimately to removal.
- Information on performance and expenditure must be accurate and timely but not overelaborate. Requests for excessively elaborate systems are often a diversion and are too likely to bring disappointment and disillusion. Selective, prompt, 'accurate enough' information is what is needed.
- Clinical directors should, in my view, be part-time and serve for a limited period. Otherwise they will in time lose the professional

end of the support they need. They are there to lead, not to manage. Their roles need to be clear, as do those of the other leaders in the directorate, eg the nurse manager and the business manager.

Clinical directorates are a means to an end, and that end is crucial. If they do not work we need something else, but they or the something else will need nurturing and maintenance. This book should help define the requirements for that nurturing and maintenance in the medium and long term.

DISCUSSION

Roger Williams: Do you see the emergence of trust hospitals' power as influencing the future of clinical directorates? I am referring, for instance, to trust hospitals actively intervening with respect to consultant contracts. For example, some consultants are conducting specialist clinics in general practitioner surgeries, and attempts have been made to appoint 'consultants' without reference to the Royal Colleges, and so on. We are seeing an emergence of central management with or without doctors in those initiatives.

Robert Maxwell: I think that your point is about centralisation and decentralisation within the system or within the institution. In my experience there is no steady state. There is a continuing tussle between forces for greater decentralisation and forces for greater centralisation; the tussle never really ends.

The creation of trusts has been an impetus towards substantially greater decentralisation of the provision of health care, and I hope that it is here to stay. Decentralised clinical directorates are related to the trusts as the trusts are related to the system of care. Trusts need to preserve and protect autonomy for the directorates, just as the system needs to preserve and protect autonomy for the trusts, and accept in both cases risks and mistakes.

Terence English: I agree with you that the preferred option of clinical management is the linkage between the institutional interest and the clinical interest, and you are suggesting that clinical directorates are the best, if not the only, way of achieving this, otherwise you might have what you described as a series of craft workshops, or the old European style of clinical management by a strong professor.

Some large institutions in the USA, such as the Cleveland Clinic and the Mayo Clinic, have a board of management entirely made up of clinicians who elect a chairman of the board. Although there are trustees or governors at the top, there is certainly no chief executive on that highest level. Indeed the chief executive, or the man or woman who actually manages the clinic, is at a very important but lower level, once the clinical staff have decided policy and strategy. So there is not really the same need for tight compartmentalised clinical directorates, because the clinicians are determining the way in which the clinic will operate as a whole. Institutional interests and the professional interests can be strongly linked in the way I have described. Presumably something like that could develop within a trust hospital.

Robert Maxwell: Yes, indeed. As I said, it is imperative to have a bond, hinge or bridge between the institution and its clinicians. Clinical directorates are only one way of doing that. You are correct that the Cleveland Clinic and the Mayo Clinic do that as well, in a quite different way. I am not sure that we could directly transfer to this country what they do; although I have visited one of them, I have not studied the institution sufficiently. Clinical directorates provide one kind of bridge between clinicians and management; if there are other mechanisms that work equally well, they can be used, but we must not fail to produce balance between management and clinicians.

Anthony Hopkins: The history of the Mayo Clinic is of a cooperative of clinicians who got together to earn fees and provide a first class clinical service and to share the necessary infrastructure. As such clinics continued to grow, clinicians appointed financial assistants, as Terence English says, beneath them, but such a structure is quite different from that of a salaried health service, even though clinicians employed by the Mayo Clinic are now salaried.

There is another lesson from that sort of structure. The chairman of the department of neurology of one clinic organised on these lines told me that he spends the first six weeks of each financial year seeing each of his many neurologists in order to set targets as to how many patients they need to see each week in order to keep up the income. Surely there must here be perverse incentives to inappropriate care. So there is a disadvantage in letting clinicians be too involved in financial concerns.

Stephen Griffin: In a hospital which has been trying hard for the past 18 months to get the structure of clinical directorates working, one of our big concerns is the resulting management costs. Development of the structure of clinical directorates requires proper support from business managers and from finance and personnel departments. Directorates also need secretarial support, offices and equipment, all of which consume money at a time when money is tight. So, just to add a note from the real world, there must be significant financial expenditure to achieve some of the things we have been talking about.

We have tried to devolve certain functions which are carried out centrally within my own directorate of personnel. This proves to be difficult when you are talking about 13 clinical directorates. How do you best deploy 2.5 staff who handle recruitment issues or 3.5 staff who handle our medical staffing across a 40 acre site?

Robert Maxwell: There should be no direct relationship between numbers of clinical directorates and numbers of business managers or managers. A business manager can cover several directorates. A good thing about clinical directorates is that they get institutional managers out of their central offices to work alongside clinicians where the real job is done. There are other real jobs to be done, in catering and cleaning etc, and all those would need to be dealt with in another set of 'workshops'. If there is to be real bonding, there has to be management support for the clinicians, but this does not necessarily require an enormous increase in the numbers of managers.

There is also a new interest in tracking costs, which engenders an increase in the number of administrators employed. For the time being, we could adopt crude national guidelines about charges, and have these as the transfer pricing mechanism and do away with some of the poor quality tracking of costs that is going on. The idea of competition does not necessarily have to take along with it an enormous increase in the number of administrators. However, when you compare the American system of health care with most European systems, that is where there is the biggest difference in the numbers of managers; their concerns are to do with the mechanisms of charging and costing, rather than managing the system.

A third element in our consideration following the NHS reforms concerns the salaries paid to managers. There has been a big increase. I think that the quality of those appointed varies, but at their best they are well worth the money.

David Scott: I would like to ask about the divergence between the trusts and the community and general practitioners. I suspect that in the next decade my specialty of rheumatology will largely be moving out of the inpatient arena and will be far more related to patients in the community. I see a future divergence of the needs of hospital trusts—your need to have a feeling of loyalty towards the place that employs you—from what patients actually need, which will be a far more community based service. How will these concerns be met within the clinical directorate structure?

Robert Maxwell: I do not know, but it would be a mistake if we let the present boundaries stand in the way of what makes sense for future development. In less developed countries, it often is the case that a hospital is a kind of oasis—a very busy oasis—often grossly overstretched, understaffed and underfinanced, but little aware of what is going on outside its own walls. I think that that is disastrous for the health care of such countries. The current wisdom that trusts must be based on single institutions or groups of institutions and must not include community services (because they cannot be trusted not to siphon money out of them) is potentially equally disastrous here. I believe that this point of view will have to be changed in the longer term. Until it is changed, those working within institutions need to work especially hard to try to get people to work as though the organisational boundaries were different.

Anthony Hopkins: There are of course other organisational models. One alternative might be to have not a clinically based directorate but an outpatient directorate, for example, from which the individual clinical departments bought time and use of its facilities. Not all directorates need to be specialty based.

Martin Severs: Organisational boundaries may result in perverse incentives. For example, there is no such item in the NHS data manual as a visit by an outpatient to a ward for review; therefore there is no remuneration, and the patient has to be seen less efficiently in outpatients or admitted as an inpatient for the institution to get its money. This is both perverse and stupid. The organisational boundaries may sometimes be in direct opposition to our professional concepts of decentralisation, devolution and delivery of care as far as possible in the patient's own home. We should try to influence the government to adopt a more devolved structure, not dividing trusts into buildings and community services, but providing services for people across organisational boundaries.

Robert Maxwell: Increasingly, the confines of the hospital will become irrelevant when finding the best way to shape services. Despite the current conventional wisdom of the Department of Health in not allowing joint applications for trust status between hospitals and community services, we have to find ways in which people can think and work across the interface between primary and secondary care, and with departments of social services. This need should determine the way in which we structure directorates and the way in which we structure the tasks of management. After all, management mechanisms exist to do something in the real world.

Many people, when they first get involved on a management course, fail to recognise the extent to which they already have a great deal of management experience. They expect some sort of instruction in the classic medical mould, such as a new set of facts to learn, which they can then go off and apply. But management is not actually like that at all; it is about surviving in turmoil.

Michael Rudolf: A common theme in our discussion has been how one gets the interests of the institution to coincide with those of individual clinicians or individual departments. Clinical directorates must have some control over their income as well as their expenditure. It seems entirely logical that the answer to both of those problems is that clinical directors must get involved in negotiations with purchasers.

In our own trust we encourage any clinical director—indeed any individual clinician should he or she so wish—to meet with at least our larger purchasing health authorities. This does, however, assume a degree of sophistication amongst purchasers that in my experience so far just does not exist. Even in dealing with fund-holding general practitioners, there is a degree of optimism or unrealism about what they think they can purchase.

We have considered the needs for the training and development of clinical directors, but purchasers are at present, from my experience, totally unaware of what we as clinical directors wish to do and wish to offer.

Anthony Hopkins: Any trust that sold clinical services to purchasers without involving the clinical directors of the services it was going to sell would be heading for disaster. Is it a widespread practice that someone will sell your services, like a prostitute, without asking you?

Tony White: We were not involved in the formulation of the contracts in my health district, and it took me eighteen months to obtain a copy. Eventually I obtained one from a fundholding general practitioner who is a personal friend. I discovered that we were regularly breaking agreements because I had no idea of what the rules were.

Andrew Frank: Contracts often do not reflect the realities of clinical practice. I can give you an illustration. One of our local hospitals declined to offer physiotherapy to one of my outpatients at a hospital nearer his home. I telephoned the purchasing authority responsible for the health care of my patient and asked whether there was a contract between his purchasing authority and the district general hospital that had declined to give physiotherapy. He affirmed this. I asked why, then, had the physiotherapy department in the middle of the year declined to offer my patient treatment. He said 'The contract is between myself (the purchaser) and the hospital to provide physiotherapy *for the patients of that hospital.*'

Ian Williams: For regional specialties, contracting is already a nightmare. My own neuroscience directorate has 12 district health authorities with which we have to negotiate and write contracts each year. At present we have 40 general practitioner fundholding practices, and from April there will be more than 100 general practitioner fundholders in our catchment area. We cannot possibly be involved in discussions with all those people. Furthermore, neurosciences are differently defined in different hospitals. Some of our colleagues find themselves negotiating as part of a directorate of 'specialties', ie a directorate of special surgery or special medicine; others are formed as directorates of neurosurgery and neurology together, and others as separate directorates. Whatever the organisation, at a meeting I organised I found that very few of them had been involved directly in contract negotiations. It was clear that some of those directorates needed to be redefined if they were to be concerned in the contract writing process, because they were not in a position to write contracts when they did not 'own' all the facilities that figure in the potential contracts.

Martin Severs: Contracts managers must not direct the way our contracts are driven. The fundamental role of the clinical director is to direct the strategy of the clinical service for which the directorate is responsible. If we delegate that responsibility, or if it is taken away by a contract manager, clinical directors do not have much of a role at all.

Robert Maxwell: We need to acknowledge, as with so many managerial things, that we are not in a steady state but in a state where a number of things, some of which are not very sensible, are being tried. We try to make the sensible things prevail. I would not be so worried about things being written into contracts that are a sort of boiler plate, at this stage, so long as we recognise that they have to be changed into more sensible patterns for the future.

The question of how one can relate a large number of contracts to a large number of clinical services is a real problem. We have to go back to basics and ask what we are trying to do. It is unacceptable to have a situation in which clinical directors are essentially only managing the expenditure budget and are not managing the income budget. That will not work. It might be feasible to have sessions at which the negotiators for the trust are briefed by the clinical directors as to what is acceptable to them and what is not. But it is clear that the result of that process must be one to which the clinical directors feel committed in terms of the income it will generate, what the prices will be, and what quality of service will be provided.

Colin Hardisty: The degree to which doctors want to get involved in purchasing varies enormously. Acute and elderly medicine will usually have just one major purchaser of facilities, which makes it much easier for these specialties to be involved in formulating contracts. Regional specialties have to deal with many more purchasing authorities.

Judith Riley: The best one can realistically hope for, except in rare situations where there are very few purchasers, is some kind of briefing, as Robert Maxwell suggests. Some of the horror stories could be stopped if clinical directors were to see contracts in draft form before they are finally signed; it should be possible to build that into the system to identify the worst problems.

In the longer term I hope that, like most professionally based organisations in which we need to make a bridge between the professionals and the managers, most managers of hospitals will know a lot about how medicine is practised. I also hope that it will be normal for some doctors to become full-time managers at some point in their careers. Doctoring is an unusual profession in which people do not choose, for the last ten years or so of their careers, to move full-time into management, unlike many other professions and industry in which specialists in various fields commonly end in general management. For me, the real long-term answer lies not in doctors undertaking individual contract negotiations, but in the people who do it really understanding your world.

Martin Rossor: Another problem is that it seems to be assumed that contracts reflect every clinical need the purchaser might have; in fact they do not recognise unmet need.

David Scott: Virement of budgets in my unit allows the block contracts, of which there are about 50, to vary between one specialty and another by up to 10%, in order to meet needs that are unexpected and not included in contracts. The effect of this has been radically to reduce the amount of elective surgical work that can go on. For example, patients in our district who need hip replacement but have not been waiting more than 18 months will have to wait a full 18 months until they reach the very end of the government's guidelines, because virement of the orthopaedic budget has occurred to pay for acute medical cases. So the whole concept of contracting and accurately adjusting work within a planned budget is undermined.

Anthony Hopkins: I am aware of the initiatives of Trent and Mersey regions in developing model contracts in relation to lung cancer, for example. If, in this example, the British Thoracic Society and the Faculty of Medical Oncology could contribute to their formulation, there would be powerful incentives for maintaining good standards of clinical practice by ensuring that such clinical guidelines formed the basis for the relevant contracts.

Colin Hardisty: Guidelines for good clinical practice, or practice protocols, are becoming part of quality measures within contracts. Barnsley health authority, for example, on which I serve, now specifies that clinical protocols are in place within directorates.

Tony White: I would like to return to the point about the relationship between central management and clinical directorates. One of the key issues there is the devolvement of authority. Some hospitals have very successfully devolved authority to clinical directors, and some have not. Has anyone any experience of how you get central management within a hospital to devolve authority so that we can have successful clinical directorates?

Robert Maxwell: It relates to an earlier point I made when talking about a hinge or a bridge or a bond between professional activity and general management. I see a necessary bond between the directorate and the institution as a two-way bond by which directorates can influence and shape the strategy for the institution as a whole. Directorates must be sufficiently powerful within the institution to ensure that there are sensible rules for delegation of authority to the directorates. Equally, there must be a sensible tension the other way to ensure that in matters of resource allocation, for example, the resources are allocated between competing bids in a way that does not simply give particularly powerful consultants their way. The directorates, collectively, need to be powerful in the management of the institution as a whole. These needs must be considered when planning the number of directorates. Whereas the current trend is towards more directorates, which makes sense for the planning of services and for seeing services as strategic medical business units, there nevertheless has to be a way in which directorates are grouped so that they can influence the institution as a whole.

10 | Summary and conclusions

Anthony Hopkins
Director, Research Unit,
Royal College of Physicians

In Chapter 9, Robert Maxwell makes it clear how there has to be some kind of hinge or bridge between the running of an institution, such as a hospital, and the independent professionals working within the institution. Clinical directorates are just one way of building that bridge. He points out that, without such a bridge or bond, health professionals will be working in an institution but not as part of it—a situation that no publicly funded organisation could continue for long—or, alternatively, health professionals will in effect be paid to pursue the policies of the institutions. As Robert Maxwell points out, either of these alternatives is 'bad news'.

We must recognise that the health care system must be responsive to users' needs. In whatever way we manage clinical practice, this is the pre-eminent requirement.

Mole and Dawson[31] point out, as have others in our discussions, that the managerial authority of clinical directors rests on the acceptance of the legitimacy of their role by their clinical colleagues and other health professionals. Our discussions underline the need for clinical directors to maintain a clinical focus in order to maintain their credibility and ensure the management of a clinical service. A distinction has been drawn (see page 4) in relation to managing a service rather than managing people. The primary aim of a clinical directorate must be to achieve the best possible outcome for the health care interventions provided by the personnel of the directorate within resources currently available. A focus on clinical audit is therefore another responsibility of clinical directors. Although supported by business managers (Chapter 5), a clinical director will need to take decisions relating to the needs of purchasers, contracts, budgets, clinical activity and outcome, hiring and firing of personnel, and indeed all the other activities—in many cases quite a considerable business.

We have considered but not resolved, many aspects of the role of clinical directorates:

- How can one give proper care to managing a clinical directorate without cutting back too far on clinical work which will remain the principal future activity of most clinical directors?
- How large should directorates be? Alternatively, how many directorates should there be in a unit?
- Should medical advisory structures, similar to Cogwheel divisions or medical staff committees, carry on in addition to the directorate structure?
- How long should be the contracts of employment of clinical directors?
- What should be the available exits for clinical directors? How many will wish to go on into more general management, and how many to return to more focused clinical activity?
- How can we attract clinicians to become clinical directors? How can we make the whole job more attractive?
- What is the most effective and economical way of training clinical directors? Who should be trained?
- How far down should budgets be devolved?
- How do we resolve the tension between the desire of a clinician to do his or her very best for an individual patient, and the volume and price contracts by which directorates are now driven?
- How can we help motivate staff to achieve changes that are not necessarily their own priorities?
- How do we resolve tensions between the professional responsibilities of nurses and the clinical directorates in which they work, and the hierarchical nursing organisation of the unit, which may have different professional views related to skill mix and so on? Equally, how do business managers resolve their mixed loyalties to the directorate and to central management?
- Who should appraise business managers, and what promotion prospects should they have? What are their opportunities for promotion into other aspects of general management?
- How much writing of internal contracts is necessary? As there are no internal competitors for such contracts, clinical directors can have little say in the quality of service provided. However, if there are explicit internal contracts, clinical directors may be able to show to general management overall inefficiencies within the unit.
- How does a clinical director review the performance of his or her fellow consultants and other members of staff?
- How best does one change the practice of doctors and other health professionals if clinical audit reveals inefficient care?
- How can the need for a big employer, such as a unit's central

management, to have an overall personnel strategy be reconciled with the smaller scale personnel requirement of a clinical directorate?

Opinions on, if not firm answers to, all these points can be found within the earlier chapters of this book.

Colleagues at the workshop were firm in some of their overall conclusions as to what clinical directors need:

- Credibility
- Accurate job descriptions
- Adequate additional financial remuneration or other non-monetary rewards
- Adequate support from a business manager
- Adequate administrative support and office space located close to the directorate's service activity
- Adequate training
- A period of organisational stability
- A wider recognition that responsibility and authority must be coterminous.
- Better budgetary information. Conversely, clinical directors have the responsibility of providing information, through clinical audit, to management in terms of clinical activity and in relation to the quality of the work they are doing. Audit should be directed towards the outcomes of the directorate's service, and not at the outcomes of interventions by individual health care professionals. For example, audit of the management of patients with stroke would be meaningless without the outcomes of interventions by physiotherapists and nurses, as well as by physicians.
- More involvement in decisions related to purchasing
- An open directorate structure, so that staff at all levels within the directorate can feel that they are contributing, that their contribution is recognised, and that their own professional needs are taken into consideration
- Freedom to determine how best to use the skills available. For example, nurse practitioners might take over some of the responsibilities of junior doctors, and less skilled nurses some of the duties currently performed by those with higher skills.
- Recognition by central management that a clinical director may not be immediately available for a business meeting with central management owing to some clinical activity. In turn, tighter agendas and better organisation of meetings would, in the view of members of the workshop, save much fruitless discussion.

- A clear exit from being a clinical director back to clinical or research work or, for some, to general management.

In many ways, I believe that we can be optimistic about the future. The bond or bridge about which Robert Maxwell writes in Chapter 9 has been already largely built. The suspicion of clinicians and managers about each others' motives, which was characteristic of life in many hospitals in the late 1970s and early 1980s, has largely disappeared. Both accept that they have different professional skills but are working to a common good. Clinical directorates are one way of linking these efforts, but the workshop from which this book is derived, and this book, underline just how much remains to be done to ensure that they become better founded.

References

1. Ministry of Health. *First report of the Joint Working Party on the Organisation of Medical Work in Hospitals* (Chairman: Sir George Godber). London: HMSO, 1967.
2. Department of Health and Social Security. *Sharing resources for health in England.* Report of the Resource Allocation Working Party. London: Department of Health, 1976.
3. *NHS and Community Care Act 1990.* London: HMSO, 1990.
4. Department of Health and Social Security. *NHS management inquiry* (Leader of inquiry: Roy Griffiths). London: DHSS, 1983.
5. Department of Health and Social Security. *Health services management: implementation of the NHS management inquiry report.* Health circular HC(84)13. London: DHSS 1983.
6. Audit Commission. *The virtue of patients: making best use of ward nursing resources.* London: HMSO, 1991.
7. Department of Health. *Working for patients.* Cm. 555. London: HMSO, 1989.
8. *The patient's charter.* London: HMSO, 1991.
9. Audit Commission. *Lying in wait.* London: HMSO, 1991.
10. Disken S, Dixon M, Halpern S, Shocket G. *Models of clinical management.* London: Institute of Health Services Management, 1990.
11. Institute of Health Services Management. *Individual performance review in the NHS.* A report by the IHSM for the NHS Management Executive. London: IHSM, 1991.
12. Salvage J. *The politics of nursing.* London: Heinemann Nursing, 1985.
13. United Kingdom Central Council. *Code of professional conduct for the nurse, midwife and health visitor.* London: UKCC, 1984.
14. Greenhalgh & Co Ltd. *Nurse management system—release 6.* Macclesfield: Health Care Management Consultants, 1991.
15. Greenhalgh & Co Ltd. (in conjunction with North West Thames, North Western, Trent, Mersey and Wessex RHAs). *Using information in managing the nursing resource.* Macclesfield: Greenhalgh, 1991.
16. Jenkins-Clarke S, Carr-Hill R. *Nursing workload measures and case-mix: an investigation of the reliability and validity of nursing workload measures.* York: Centre for Health Economics, 1991.
17. McClure M, Poulin M, Sovie M, Wandelt MA. *Magnet hospitals: attraction and retention of professional nurses.* Kansas City: American Nurses Association, 1983.
18. Dean D. What makes a magnet? *Health Service Journal* 1991; 101: 18–9.
19. Shenton H, Hamm C. How to retain nurses. *The Professional Nurse* 1988: 360–2.
20. Scope of practice. *The Nursing Times* 1992; **88:** 26–30.
21. Lohr K. *A strategy for quality assurance.* Vol 1. Washington DC: National Academy Press, 1990.
22. Maxwell RJ. Quality assessment in health. *British Medical Journal* 1984: 288: 1470–2.
23. Donabedian A. *The definition of quality and approaches to its assessment.* Michigan: Health Administration Press, 1980.
24. NHS Management Executive. *Clinical audit in HCHS: allocation of funds.* EL(93)34, 1993–4.
25. Berwick DM, Bunker JP. Enthoven A. Quality management in the NHS: the doctor's role – II. *British Medical Journal* 1992; **304:** 304–8.
26. Wraith Casey Management Consultants. *Implementing clinically based management: getting organisational change underway.* Droitwich: Wraith Casey Management Consultants, 1992.
27. Wraith Casey Management Consultants. *New management in evolution.* Droitwich: Wraith Casey Management Consultants, 1992.
28. Jack Lane Associates. *Evaluation of management development for hospital consultants.* Ware: Jack Lane Associates, 1991.
29. The Times. *Performance figures show variable quality of NHS care.* 26 April 1993.
30. Hopkins A. Doubts over hospital league tables. *The Times,* 30 April 1993.
31. Mole V, Dawson S. Pole to pole – Special report on clinical management. *Health Service Journal* 1993; 103: 33–4.

Further Bibliography

Appleby JL. Why doctors must grapple with health economics. *British Medical Journal* 1987; **294:** 326.

Brider P. Patient focussed care. *American Journal of Nursing* 1992; September: 26–33.

British Association of Medical Managers. British Medical Association. Institute of Health Services Management, Royal College of Nursing. *Managing clinical services: a consensus statement of principles for effective clinical management.* London: Institute of Health Services Management, 1993.

Bunch C. Developing a hospital information strategy: a clinician's view. *British Medical Journal* 1992; **304:** 1036.

Carle N. *Managing for health result.* Papers from a King's Fund international seminar. London: King Edward's Hospital Fund for London, 1990.

Chantler C. How to be a manager. *British Medical Journal* 1989; **298:** 1505–8.

Chantler C. Management and information. *British Medical Journal* 1992; **304:** 632–5.

Costain D, ed. *The future of acute services: doctors as managers.* London: King's Fund Centre for Health Services Development, 1990.

Davies P. IPR is put through its paces and found wanting. *Health Service Journal* 1991; 101: 13.

Delbecq AL, Gill SL. Justice as a prelude to teamwork in medical centers. *Health Care Management Review* 1989; **10:** 53–9.

Department of Health and Social Security and Welsh Office. *Patients first.* Consultative paper on the structure and management of the National Health Service in England and Wales. London: HMSO, 1979.

Department of Health and Social Security. *Resource management (management budgeting) in health authorities.* HN(86)34. DHSS, 1986.

Drummond M. *Incentives for health care professionals.* Paper prepared for King's Fund meeting on the 40th anniversary of the NHS. London: King Edward's Hospital Fund for London, 1988.

Ellwood PM. Outcomes management: a technology of patient experience. Shattuck Lecture. *New England Journal of Medicine* 1988; **318:** 1549–56.

Fitzgerald L. Made to measure. *Health Service Journal* 1991: 101: 24–5.

Fitzgerald L. This year's model. *Health Service Journal* 1991: 101: 26—27.

Ham C, Hunter DJ. *Managing clinical activity in the NHS.* London: King's Fund Institute, 1988.

Heyssel RM, Gaintner JR. Kues IW, Jones AA, Lipstein SH. Decentralised management in a teaching hospital. *New England Journal of Medicine* 1984; **310:** 1477–80.

Hopkins A. *Measuring the quality of medical care.* London: Royal College of Physicians, 1990.

Maxwell RJ. *Shaping the NHS for the 1990s.* London: King Edward's Hospital Fund for London, 1989.

Maxwell RJ, Morrison V, eds. *Working with people.* Papers from a King's Fund international seminar. London: King Edward's Hospital Fund for London, 1983.

Social Services Committee. *The future of the National Health Service.* Session 1987–1988, 5th report. HC613. London: HMSO, 1988.

Steele B. Clinical information systems. *British Journal of Healthcare Computing* 1989; **6:** 25–6.

Stoeckle JD, Reiser SJ. The composite organisation of hospital work: balancing professional and administrative responsibilities. *Annals of Internal Medicine* 1992; **116:** 407–13.

West PA. *Understanding the NHS: a question of incentives.* London: King Edward's Hospital Fund for London, 1988.

White T. *Management for clinicians.* London: Edward Arnold, 1993.

Young DW. Clinical computing systems; their slow introduction. *Postgraduate Medical Journal* 1990; **66:** 333–5.

APPENDIX 1
Key tasks for clinical directors

The tasks are drawn from the Middlesex Business School's evaluation of management development for hospital consultants[28] and are reproduced with permission.

A clinical director should be able to perform the following tasks:

- Resolve effectively any conflict arising from the combining of the traditional consultant role and that of clinical director
- Marry the activities of the medical audit process with managerial policies to deliver a quality service to patients
- Enact effectively the managerial relationship between him(her)self and consultants, whilst maintaining good relations and morale (yours and the consultants')
- Maintain effective and constructive relationships with other clinical directors/medical managers and managers within the wider organisation
- Adopt a strategic perspective
- Develop appropriate and workable policies for the running of the unit
- Produce an accurate budget for the directorate 6, 12 and 24 months (or more) ahead
- Utilise financial concepts such as direct and indirect costs, depreciation, full costing, marginal costing, profit and loss accounts, and revenue and capital expenditure
- Distinguish between management and financial accounting statements
- Negotiate successfully and agree the budget with the general manager
- Monitor actual performance against budgeted performance
- Control activities in the light of differences between planned and actual performance
- Verify the accuracy of a manpower plan
- Develop appropriate job descriptions
- Develop personnel specifications
- Make valid and accurate assessments of people
- Motivate key staff to achieve agreed performance objectives, and beyond
- Accept responsibility for the performance of all the people in the directorate, and provide the guidance and leadership necessary for effective management

- Recognise the different abilities of team members and build well motivated and effective teams
- Chair an effective meeting, lead a discussion group, and conduct a team briefing
- Monitor staff performance and make valid assessments taking into account situational factors and personal abilities
- Conduct an effective review of an individual's performance which leaves the person appraised with agreed personal and performance objectives and motivated towards attaining them
- Handle a disciplinary or grievance issue brought by a member of the directorate staff
- Identify room for improvements in services to patients
- Negotiate and agree the introduction of change
- Implement and evaluate the effects of change
- Deal effectively with staff who are perhaps defensive and resentful about the changes taking place around them
- Cope with staff who actively may resist change, keeping within the organisation's grievance and disciplinary procedures
- Obtain and evaluate information to aid decision making
- Recommend changes and/or improvements in information technology equipment to facilitate the supply and quality of information
- Distinguish between data and information
- Provide the leadership qualities to establish and maintain that role
- Manage personal emotions and stress
- Maintain self-confidence and personal drive
- Effectively manage personal time and organisation
- See tasks through to completion, irrespective of obstacles and setbacks
- Maintain flexibility and openness to new ideas and change

APPENDIX 2
An organisational development checklist for clinical directorate management teams

The questions are based on the Wraith Casey report 'New management in evolution'[26] and are reproduced with permission.

Overall management practice

- Have we truly agreed the philosophy of the directorate and operational rules and published and disseminated them?
- Are objectives and aims clear, corporately owned and well published?
- What is our corporate 'vision'?
- Do we have an organisational development plan that enables us to achieve our vision?
- Do we have jointly owned and agreed strategies (eg operational, communications, staff development and training)?
- Are mechanisms for reviewing and adjusting the above in place and effective?
- Is our management structure the best option? Does it allow true representation and participation?
- Are we clear about our separate and corporate roles and responsibilities and are they well demonstrated and communicated to staff?
- Are we and everyone in the directorate clear about who makes decisions about what?
- Are we clear about how we will effectively monitor the direction, performance and climate of the directorate? Have we told everyone else who should know?
- Who needs to relate to people and issues outside the directorate? How do we ensure this happens effectively?
- What is our system of review of personal and directorate performance and how is this working?
- How do we prepare for reviews and how do we act on issues raised?

Teamwork

- How well do we work together?
- Are we clear about our individual strengths and contributions?
- Do we support and complement each other?

- How are we developing individually and as a team? What more can we do? What changes should we make?
- How are we using teamwork within the directorate?
- How active are we in encouraging, supporting and developing it?
- Whom in particular can we develop further as team leaders?
- What more should we be doing?

Communication

- Do we share the right information at the right time?
- Is written communication effective?
- Do we meet too often or not often enough?
- Do we have clear aims for our meetings?
- Do our meetings achieve their aims?
- Do we listen to and hear each other?
- Do people receive sufficient, relevant information?
- Are there sufficient open channels of communication to encourage people to talk to each other 'up and down' through the directorate?
- Are directorate meetings and written communications effective?
- What else is needed?
- Are mechanisms in place for effective inter- and intra-professional communication?
- How aware are we of what staff think and feel on different issues and how can they express these views?
- Are external communications sufficient and efficient (eg trust board, hospital council, other directorates, community units, patients, families, the public)?

Decision making

- What decisions does the directorate make and not make? Do we need to change anything?
- Are decisions timely?
- Do we communicate, monitor and review decisions?
- Do the right people make them? Are they delegated to the appropriate level?
- Do staff know what decisions are made, why and what are their implications?
- Are we clear when full consultation, debate or consensus is necessary?

Leadership style

- What is our style? Is it corporate? Is it what we want? Is it

working? Is it compatible with our philosophy?
- Do we respect each other and other professionals? Do we respect, encourage and reward particular skills and contributions sufficiently?
- Do we encourage mutual support and learning?
- Are we approachable, available and responsive?
- Do we listen to people?
- Do we and are we seen to set the style and pace of the directorate?
- Do we delegate and then empower people sufficiently to deal with additional responsibility?
- Do we hold people accountable in a constructive way?
- Do we confront disrespect, obstructive behaviour, conflict and difficulty in a constructive way?
- Do we deal with bad practice appropriately?

Culture and climate

- Do we have a corporate directorate identity?
- Are people proud to work here?
- Is this a positive, creative and satisfying place to work?
- Is success rewarded?
- Do we encourage and support new developments?
- Do people feel safe to take risks?
- Does change threaten people inappropriately? If so, how can we instil change as a positive experience?
- Do we encourage good leadership? How can we groom potential leaders?
- Do we encourage constructive criticism and feedback?
- Do people feel safe to express negative and contrary views?
- Do we discourage inappropriate bureaucracy?
- Do we give credit where credit is due?
- Do we delegate to people with appropriate skill rather than to people in a certain hierarchical position?

APPENDIX 3
Clinical directorates: worries, key factors for success and advantages of clinical directorates.

These points were made by a subgroup of 40 doctors 'brainstorming' at the joint conference sponsored by the British Association of Medical Managers, the British Medical Association, the Institute of Health Services Management and the Royal College of Nursing on 'Managing clinical services' held in London, 23–24 September 1992.

What worries us

- Management is not decentralised
- Central management may fail to 'let go' of decision making
- Loss of clinical time is excessive
- Decentralised management is a ruse for devolving financial responsibility
- Clinical directors have responsibility without power, that is without control of budget
- Clinicians will have to carry the can for problems outside their control
- Weaker specialties may lose resources to the stronger
- Potential exists for conflict between the clinical director and his or her colleagues
- Financial information is insufficiently robust to allow good management
- Clinical directors have insufficient management training

Some key factors for success

- Leadership skills, and the ability to manage change
- Mutual trust between the clinical director and other clinicians, and between clinicians and management
- Commitment from most of the medical staff
- Provision of adequate managerial, financial and secretarial support; the clinical director needs to be involved in selecting his or her primary support team
- Provision of accurate information, and adequate information and communication systems; clinicians may help provide central

management with relevant financial information from the bottom up, and may spot absurdities which initially seem financially sound
- Support from spouse
- Sufficient time
- Ability to move resources according to current need
- Team approach
- Appropriate financial or other incentives
- Presence within a decentralised group of a consultant ready, willing and able to lead and manage the directorate
- Willing cooperation of nursing and management
- Adequate education of doctors and managers about each others' capabilities and responsibilities.

Some advantages of clinical directorates

- Encouragement of loyalty and commitment from all grades of staff and bonding between groups: nurses, doctors, physiotherapists, clerks etc
- Opportunity for doctors to be 'in control'
- 'We' (doctors and managers together) replaces 'them and us'
- Quicker decisions and improved patient care
- Greater awareness of the utilisation of resources